PUBLIC HEALTH IN THE 21ST CENTURY

COMMUNITY HEALTH WORKERS

EMERGING ROLE AND INTERVENTION OUTCOMES

(WITH ACCOMPANYING CD-ROM)

Public Health in the 21st Century

Additional books in this series can be found on Nova's website under the Series tab.

Additional e-books in this series can be found on Nova's website under the e-book tab.

PUBLIC HEALTH IN THE 21ST CENTURY

COMMUNITY HEALTH WORKERS

EMERGING ROLE AND INTERVENTION OUTCOMES

(WITH ACCOMPANYING CD-ROM)

CECILIA HODGES
EDITOR

nova publishers
New York

NOTICE TO THE READER

Additional color graphics may be available in the e-book version of this book.

Library of Congress Cataloging-in-Publication Data

ISBN: 978-1-63485-060-5

Published by Nova Science Publishers, Inc. † New York

CONTENTS

Preface

A community health worker (CHW) is a frontline public health worker who, as a member of the community, has the potential to deliver cost-effective, high quality, and culturally competent health services within team-based care models. This book reviews select health services research findings on community health worker utilization that are relevant to U.S. policymakers and considers the key challenges to fully realizing the potential for CHWs to improve health care delivery.

This book is accompanied by a CD-ROM which includes appendices A through E for Chapter Two, *Outcomes of Community Health Worker Interventions*.

In: Community Health Workers
Editor: Cecilia Hodges
ISBN: 978-1-63485-060-5

Chapter 1

COMMUNITY HEALTH WORKERS: ROLE AND OPPORTUNITIES IN HEALTH CARE DELIVERY SYSTEM REFORM*

John E. Snyder

This report reviews select health services research findings on Community Health Worker (CHW) utilization that are relevant to U.S. policymakers and considers the key challenges to fully realizing the potential for CHWs to improve health care delivery.

Main Findings

- Community Health Workers (CHWs) are an emerging group of health professionals that have recently drawn increased national attention because of their potential to deliver cost-effective, high quality, and culturally competent health services within team-based care models.
- The apparent benefits of integrating CHWs into health care teams seem to depend on context. The strongest evidence of these benefits supports utilizing CHWs to deliver certain specific, high-value, preventive services – focused on reducing risk factors for cardiovascular disease and other chronic conditions – to low-income, minority, or other underserved populations.
- Despite growing interest in engaging CHWs in national delivery system reform efforts, there are several uncertainties about how to best proceed with this. Questions remain around standardizing CHW training, certification, and licensure; establishing strong economic and other evidence to support their use; and securing reimbursement for their services to ensure financial sustainability of CHW programs.

---

* This is an edited, reformatted and augmented version of a report issued by the U.S. Department of Health and Human Services, Office of the Assistant Secretary for Planning and Evaluation, January 2016.

INTRODUCTION

Health care reform activities since the 2010 passage of the Affordable Care Act have resulted in significant and innovative shifts in health service delivery and reimbursement – with an overall movement towards increased value, coordination, and accountability in care. Accompanying these changes, many of the traditional roles and services of providers such as physicians, nurses, and other health care workers have expanded and evolved. In addition, some emerging, new occupations are playing an increasing role in patient-centered medical homes (PCMHs) and other team-based models for health care delivery [1]. Although community health workers (CHWs) have been embedded in community-based outreach programs for decades, significant national policy interest is emerging for this the occupation due to the potential ability of CHWs to improve health care access, service delivery, and care coordination, and to provide enhanced value in health care investments [2].

Although there is some variability in how the U.S. Department of Labor [3] and other organizations [4] define a "Community Health Worker," a CHW is typically a frontline public health worker who is a trusted member of, and/or has an unusually close understanding of, the community served. This trusting relationship enables the worker to serve as a link between community members and needed health and social services within their community. CHWs hold a unique position within an often rigid health care system in that they can be flexible and creative in responding to specific individual and community needs. Their focus is often on the social, rather than the medical, determinants of health – addressing the socioeconomic, cultural practices, and organizational barriers affecting wellness and access to care [5] CHWs are known by numerous names in their communities and in the health literature, including Promotores de Salud, Community Health Advisors, and related titles [6, 7, 8] reflecting their widely variable roles and responsibilities. This variability can present a challenge for demonstrating their value through outcomes research and for attempts to standardize CHW educational pathways, certification, and reimbursement [9, 10]

This report reviews select health services research findings on CHW utilization that are relevant to U.S. policymakers and considers the key challenges to fully realizing and quantifying the potential for CHWs to improve health care delivery. Although not intended to be a comprehensive and critical analysis of the full body of research around CHWs, this paper builds on information from a number of recent reports from across the Department of Health and Human Services (HHS) – including a 2009 systematic review by the Agency for Healthcare Research and Quality (AHRQ) [11], a 2014 evidence assessment published by the Centers for Disease Control and Prevention (CDC) [12], a 2015 CDC policy brief on CHW interventions for chronic disease management [13], and a 2015 summary of findings by the CDC-supported Community Preventive Services Task Force on cardiovascular disease interventions [14]. This material is supplemented with select additions from the primary health literature and reports by health policy research organizations.

ROLES IN HEALTH CARE DELIVERY

The primary goals for deploying CHWs in health care teams are to increase access, deliver screening and preventive services, and improve system navigation, care coordination, and disease management outcomes through education and other approaches (Table 1). The unique strength of CHWs is their ability to develop rapport with patients and other community members due to shared culture, community residence, and life experiences. They are also able to enhance the cultural and linguistic appropriateness of care and help to counteract factors such as social exclusion, poverty, and marginalization [15, 16] As such, and aside from the objectives for deploying them from the health system perspective, an important component of the CHW occupational identity can be to advocate for the socioeconomic, environmental, and political rights of their communities [17].

The ability of CHWs to relate to patients can enable them to elicit candid information and collect more accurate clinical data than other health care workers [18]. Additionally, their patient- and family-centered approaches can improve the comprehension of and adherence to provider instructions [19, 20]. Expertise in conducting outreach positions some CHWs as a resource for navigating health insurance options and successfully enrolling people in Medicaid or Marketplace plans [21, 22]. CHW work at the interface between health systems and the community has the potential to reduce the inappropriate use of high-cost health services, such as emergency room visits for primary care health needs and unnecessary hospital readmissions [23].

CHWs are most often deployed to improve outcomes in communities with high levels of health disparities or a disproportionate prevalence of chronic disease [24]. One major goal of delivery system reform is to respond strategically to the growing national prevalence of multiple chronic conditions by improving care coordination. By 2020, 157 million people in the have one chronic condition and 81 million to have multiple chronic conditions [25]. The growing national burden of chronic illness is borne to a greater extent by minority and low-income populations, who experience poorer health outcomes [26]. For example, the likelihood that non-Hispanic black adults in the U.S. will die prematurely of cardiovascular or cerebrovascular disease is at least 50 percent greater than for non-Hispanic white adults [27], and infant mortality rates for non-Hispanic blacks are more than double those of non-Hispanic whites [28] Diabetes is more prevalent in non-Hispanic black adults, those with Hispanic ethnicity, adults with lower incomes, and those without a college education than in other segments of the population [29].

Such health inequities have large individual, community, and economic impacts. According to a 2009 study by the Joint Center for Political and Economic Studies, the combined additional costs to the national economy of health inequalities and premature death of minority groups in the U.S. were estimated to be total approximately $1.24 trillion from 2003–2006 [30]. This is likely due to a combination of both direct expenses from delivering health care to a sicker and more disadvantaged population and indirect costs attributed to employment-related factors and premature mortality (e.g., lower productivity, lost wages and tax revenues, leave to deal with avoidable family illnesses). Strategies that can effectively address social determinants of health and counteract health inequities experienced by vulnerable patient populations will have significant societal and economic benefits for the nation. Given their strong bonds with communities and ability to facilitate access, coordination, capacity building, and service delivery, CHWs are seen as one potential solution for achieving these aims.

Table 1. Major Roles for Community Health Workers in the U.S. Health System

Model	Function	Examples of goals/activities
Lay Health Worker/ Promotora de Salud	Address social determinants of health and risk factors for chronic diseases	• screening for behavioral and other risk factors (e.g., hypertension) for chronic conditions (e.g., cardiovascular disease) • encouraging self-reporting and facilitating self-management around health behaviors (e.g., smoking cessation, exercise) • offering social support and informal counseling
Health Educator	Provide education services	• delivering individual or group education • encouraging adherence and compliance with treatments and medications
Outreach and Enrollment Agent	Increase care access	• identifying individuals and families eligible for medical services • assisting in the application for medical services
Team-Based Care Member	Collaboratively provide direct health services with medical professionals	• improving care coordination • providing patient support when paired with licensed health care providers (physicians, nurses)
Care Coordinator and Navigator	Assist in care coordination for those with complex health conditions	• monitoring and follow-up (appointment reminders, home visits) • assisting individuals and families in navigating complex medical service systems and processes
Community Organizer and Capacity Builder	Share social, cultural, and economic characteristics with community	• supporting community development □ serving as liaisons between the community and health care systems • advocating for patients and communities, promoting community action • building community support for new activities

Sources: Community Preventive Services Task Force (http://www.thecommunity guide.org/cvd/CHW.html).

Rural Assistance Center (https://www.raconline.org/communityhealth).

Table 2. Community Health Worker employment – facts and figures

Number of CHWs in the U.S., 2012	99,400
Projected percent change in employment from 2012 to 2022 (average for all occupations is 11%)	21%
Paid versus volunteer	Up to 40% may work as unpaid volunteers
Median pay, 2012	$41,830 annually or $21.11 per hour
States with the highest CHW employment level	• California • Illinois • Texas • New York • Florida

Sources: Bureau of Labor Statistics (2012) and National Community Health Worker Advocacy Survey (2014).

CHW Training and Credentialing

CHWs are distinct from the other members of health care teams in that they are hired primarily for their understanding of the populations and communities they serve rather than for expertise or credentials obtained through formal health education [31]. As such, they are traditionally trained after hiring to use their personal perspectives and experiences to link patients within their communities to services. According to one 2014 survey, up to 40 percent of all CHWs nationally may work as unpaid volunteers (Table 2) [32]. Thus CHWs differ from most other health care workers who usually have prolonged training in clinical care and formal qualifications prior to employment and who are generally paid for their services.

The extent to which CHWs are trained to perform their roles and whether or how they become certified or licensed to deliver care varies greatly from state to state, based on state and organizational licensure requirements. Several states have passed legislation identifying CHW training that could eventually be used as a prerequisite for reimbursement, while many other states are at various stages of the policy development process. For example, in Minnesota, a CHW state-standardized curriculum is offered through the postsecondary educational system [33]. CHWs receive a certificate on completion of this curriculum that qualifies them to enroll for reimbursement under the state Medicaid program, one of only two established reimbursement models for CHWs within public insurance programs to date in which CHWs are reimbursed directly [34]. By contrast, the state of New Mexico has no statute regarding CHWs but their Department of Health maintains a robust CHW advisory board that recommends certification standards and training, and which has disciplinary authority [35].

Legislative tracking of CHW training and certification requirements is performed by the Association of State and Territorial Health Officials (ASTHO). As of October 2015, ASTHO reports [36] that:

- Six states (FL, MA, NM, OH, OR, TX) have laws or regulations which establish CHW certification program requirements.

- Two states (IL, MD) have statutes creating a CHW advisory board, taskforce, or workgroup to establish certification program requirements.
- Seven states (IN, MS, NE, NV, NY, SC, WA) have no laws in place but have state-led training or certification programs.
- Two states (AK, MN) have established Medicaid payments for services provided by a certified CHW.
- One state (FL), which already provides some CHW credentialing guidelines, has reintroduced legislation (that did not move forward in the prior legislative session) to define the duties of a CHW and establish a voluntary process by which a department-approved third-party credentialing entity may grant a credential to an eligible individual.
- The remaining 33 states and the District of Columbia have not taken or introduced regulatory or legislative action around CHW education, certification requirements, or establishing Medicaid payments for CHW-provided services.

Although flexibility in responding to specific individual and community needs is considered to be a key strength of CHWs, the lack of consistent, standardized CHW educational pathways and the varying scopes of practice observed across different CHW roles are likely reasons why more universal credentialing standards have not been developed [37]. This is a well-recognized barrier for CHWs in achieving greater respect among the other health care professions, improving their compensation and working conditions, increasing their job stability and portability, and better integrating them into the U.S. health system [38, 39, 40] In addition, as credentialing is often a critical component for insurance reimbursement, this lack of standardization may limit the potential for CHW service reimbursement by both public and private insurance plans [41]. To this end, the focus of the Community Health Worker Core Consensus (C3) Project is to help advance consensus in the CHW field around local, state, and national training curricula and practice guidelines for the occupation [42]. On the other hand, many CHWs have expressed concerns that standardized credentialing could create job entry barriers for the best-suited CHW candidates, such as members of diverse, low-income communities who may additionally have language barriers [43].

A National Profile of CHWs

In 2014, the Arizona Prevention Research Center of the University of Arizona, working through a cooperative agreement with the CDC, collected information from 1,767 CHWs from 45 states and four U.S. territories through the online National Community Health Worker Advocacy Survey [44]. This research project examined demographic information, training, work environment, job-related roles and activities, and target populations served. The voluntary, and potentially non-representative survey was distributed online to CHWs through local, state, and national organizations and was available in three different languages (English, Spanish, and Korean).

Results of the survey showed that CHWs were more likely to be female (89 percent) with an average age of 45. The range of self-reported race and ethnicity roughly matched the composition of the communities served. The most common self-identified race was white (23 percent), and 45 percent of CHWs identified their ethnicity as Hispanic. Almost all had a high school diploma or equivalent, 13 percent had no college, approximately two-thirds reported at least some college education, and 14 percent held a graduate degree.

Paid CHWs (60 percent of the sample) tended to be full-time workers, whereas volunteers worked an average of 12 hours per week. Excluding volunteers, income varied but mostly ranged between $10-50,000 per year, and 78 percent reported having employer-sponsored health insurance. Site of employment varied greatly, with community-based sites (37 percent) the most common, followed by federally-qualified health centers (17 percent), hospitals (14 percent), local health departments (12 percent), and other clinics (10 percent). Consistent with medical literature and case studies, the survey found that most CHWs worked to deliver or promote preventive services (67 percent) although 36 percent reported working to increase access to health care services, and 24 percent reported working in areas related to mental and behavioral health. Many reported roles managing various common chronic diseases, such as cancer, cardiovascular disease, HIV infection, and diabetes.

Although known by a slightly different term, Community Health Representatives (CHRs) have served American Indian/Alaska Native communities in a manner similar to CHWs for several decades, and are supported by HHS through Indian Health Service (IHS) funds [45]. There are currently more than 1,700 CHRs representing 264 tribes [46, 47, 48] The National Association of Community Health Representatives (NACHR) has representatives from twelve service areas who help to shape national policies for CHRs and to identify and disseminate promising practices [49]. A 2013 NACHR survey, similar to that performed by the Arizona Prevention Research Center, collected data on CHRs, with a subsequent report [50] describing many characteristics of the CHR workforce. The IHS provides training and technical assistance to the Indian, Tribal, and Urban Facilities who utilize CHR's across the twelve service areas. In the IHS publication *Trends in Indian Health* (2014 edition) [51], the three leading activities since 2007 for CHRs were case management (23 percent), health education (14 percent), and patient care services (15 percent). CHRs received over 1.7 million referrals from community contacts and providers during that period, providing about 5.7 million client contacts to address health concerns related to diabetes mellitus (15 percent), hypertension (10 percent), other health promotion/disease prevention (10 percent), heart problems (5 percent), nutrition (4 percent), dialysis (4 percent), and other health care needs.

It is notable that utilization of CHWs within health care systems has been far more extensive internationally than it has been in the United States [52, 53]. In many other countries, CHWs are increasingly being integrated into community-based health care systems as paid, full-time health care workers. For example, the One Million Community Health Workers Campaign is training and deploying CHWs into the health systems of sub-Saharan Africa, and as many as 600,000 CHWs in India currently provide certain primary care services, such as vaccination, and are reimbursed for their work through a fee-for-service system. In parts of Europe and in Brazil, CHWs are integrated into health care teams providing maternal and child health care, mental health services, and chronic disease management.

Evidence on the Clinical Impact of CHWs

In line with the far greater extent of CHW deployment seen in other countries, much of the evidence base demonstrating CHW effectiveness in improving health care outcomes has been established internationally [54] HHS has conducted several reviews of the literature on the achieved outcomes, cost-effectiveness, and regulation of CHWs in the United States. These literature summaries and systematic reviews, performed or supported by CDC and AHRQ, seem to suggest that CHWs provide highly context-dependent benefits – with the greatest advantages seen when CHWs deliver certain specific preventive services to low-income, minority, or other underserved populations. The findings from these efforts are briefly summarized below.

In 2009, AHRQ commissioned the RTI International–University of North Carolina Evidence-based Practice Center to perform a systematic review of the health literature on the outcomes, costs, and cost-effectiveness of CHW interventions [55]. This review concluded that, while large-scale evidence on CHW effectiveness in the U.S. is lacking, there are numerous smaller studies in the literature from state and local programs or that focused on specific patient populations. From the 68 identified studies, limited evidence favored CHW interventions over control groups or alternative approaches. However the clinical context of individual studies was deemed to be important, since the most encouraging findings were from interventions focusing on low-income, minority, or other underserved populations. Relatively positive outcomes were seen when CHWs facilitated delivery of certain specific preventive services (e.g., disease prevention, asthma management, cervical cancer screening with Pap smears, and mammography screening) but not others (e.g., clinical breast examination, breast self-examination, colorectal cancer screening, chronic disease management, and most maternal and child health interventions). Such studies commonly focused on specific health or cost-effectiveness outcomes related to integrating CHWs onto health care teams to help manage chronic diseases or to deliver preventive services. This review noted that the identified studies can be limited by inadequate power and a lack of rigorous research methodology. They often use non-quantitative approaches, have null findings, may be influenced by a Hawthorne effect, or are not easily comparable to each other due to differing approaches. Therefore, this review concluded that, without further research, methodological limitations make it difficult to draw definitive conclusions from the existing body of literature in order to inform policy decisions at a national level.

A CDC report in 2014 assessed and summarized the strengths and limitations of the evidence base behind a number of chronic disease policy interventions that included CHWs. From this, the CDC determined the potential for these interventions to inform future chronic disease policy decision-making (Appendix A) [56]. The greatest potential was seen for CHW deployment onto interprofessional teams under provider supervision (nurse practitioners or physicians) for interventions focused on access, patient self-management, chronic disease management, cost reduction, and improved social outcomes. This was particularly true if CHWs were assisting patient groups with significant health disparities – such as those who were low-income, uninsured, or belonging to certain racial and ethnic minority groups (e.g., African American, Asian, Filipino, Bangladeshi, Vietnamese, and Hispanic populations).

Another CDC report summarized evidence around CHW interventions designed to prevent chronic diseases, particularly those which tend to be influenced heavily by socioeconomic factors – such as hypertension, diabetes, cancer, and asthma [57]. The clearest results were observed for patient education interventions focused on improving treatment adherence and self-management among specific patient groups based on age, race, or ethnicity. For example, there was some evidence that working with CHWs could be a cost-effective way to reduce symptoms of asthma in adolescents, for certain cancer patients to achieve more timely diagnosis and treatment, or for hypertensive patients to better adhere to medical appointments and prescribed medications.

In 2015, the CDC-supported Community Preventive Services Task Force systematically reviewed evidence from 31 research publications on prevention-focused CHW interventions targeting cardiovascular disease (CVD) risk factors, such as hypertension and dyslipidemia, in certain minority groups and underserved communities [58]. The Task Force determined that there was strong evidence across the literature base supporting the effectiveness of integrating CHWs into team-based care models, alongside physicians and nurses, to improve patient blood pressure and cholesterol levels. Some benefits were also observed for interventions focusing on health education, insurance outreach and enrollment activities, and in increasing patient health behaviors involving diet, exercise, and tobacco cessation. Little evidence was identified for CHWs improving outcomes related to health system navigation, decreasing costs, reducing hospital length of stay or readmissions, decreasing emergency room visits, or improving mortality.

Reimbursement

Providing reimbursement for CHW services is an evolving and important policy area since lack of sustainable funding remains a significant challenge to the CHW occupation [59]. The short-term grants and contracts that currently support most CHW programs potentially create unstable work prospects because funding streams are vulnerable to changes in economics, politics, and agency strategies. Reimbursement for CHW services might additionally incentivize health care systems, provider groups, and health plans to recruit, use, and retain effective CHWs to improve the quality of care delivered to their served populations. Medicaid reimbursement for CHW services is currently possible through a few different mechanisms – including leverage of the January 2014 Centers for Medicare & Medicaid Services (CMS) final rule (CMS-2334-F) on Essential Health Benefits [60, 61]. This rule gives states the new option to provide Medicaid reimbursement for preventive services recommended by, rather than provided directly by, a physician or other licensed practitioner. Hence, direct patient medical services can be furnished at the recommendation of a licensed provider by another health worker, such as a CHW, who may or may not be formally licensed by the state. As of November 2015, no states have completed this state plan amendment process to tap into this new reimbursement stream.

Additional Medicaid reimbursement mechanisms include capitation, direct reimbursement arrangements, waivers, and state support of administrative costs (see Appendix B for a more detailed discussion of this). Of these, capitation is likely the most promising as per-member, per-month payments to managed care health plans can be used to pay CHW salaries so long as this option is in accordance with the contract and both federal and state regulations [62]. Through direct reimbursement arrangements with a provider, community, or tribal organization, state Medicaid offices may opt to make CHWs a billable provider [63]. Such arrangements specify allowable reimbursement rates as well as the education, training, and certification requirements for providers. The CMS Center for Medicaid and CHIP Services (CMCS) may also match a percent of staffing and administrative expenses for state Medicaid offices and clinics to better achieve cost control, improve information technology infrastructure, and provide interpreter, outreach, and coordination services [64]. Some of these activities may include using CHWs. State-initiated waivers, such as those allowed under Section 1115 of the Social Security Act, provide opportunities for a state Medicaid program to pilot innovative, budget-neutral demonstration projects which include CHW and other services not traditionally covered by the program [65]. Many states are taking advantage of funding through "Delivery System Reform Incentive Payment" (DSRIP) initiatives, a type of Section 1115 Waiver tied to performance metrics, to promote payment and system redesign which helps them achieve statewide population health goals [66]. Complementing this, CMS launched the Medicaid Innovation Accelerator Program in 2014 with the goal of supporting states' efforts to fast-track reforms aimed at improving health care for Medicaid beneficiaries [67]. As opportunities such as DSRIP waivers and the Medicaid Innovation Accelerator Program help states move towards more integrated care for safety net populations across all delivery settings, this can be an impetus for states to consider incorporating CHWs into their health programs. And as new payment models continue to evolve toward capitated mechanisms for reimbursement or global payments, it is may be less important for CHWs to be reimbursable as a provider type or as someone who provides a specified service.

OPPORTUNITIES THROUGH THE CMS INNOVATION CENTER

The mission of the CMS Innovation Center is to foster health care transformation by developing and testing new models to pay for and deliver health services that can lower costs and improve care – and encouraging widespread adoption of models that achieve this [68]. As the focus of CHW services is often to help better manage chronic disease, improve care quality and outcomes, and decrease the overall cost of care, many care models being tested within the CMS Innovation Center demonstrations seek to leverage the strengths of CHWs. These workers are included in a number of State Innovation Model strategies (in CO, CT, DE, HI, IA, IL, MD, ME, MI, MN, OH, OR, and PA – see Appendix C) and in many of the demonstration projects that have been funded under the Center's Health Care Innovation Awards (Appendix D) [69, 70, 71, 72]. It will be important to follow the outcomes of these funded initiatives to determine if CHW interventions help achieve the CMS Innovation Center's goals, and if these health system strategies should be more widely disseminated across the nation.

CONCLUSIONS

Health care delivery system reform efforts are stimulating movement away from traditional, fee for service-based reimbursement towards newer payment models that focus on value, quality, care coordination, and accountability. Integrating CHWs into care teams may be one potential strategy to further facilitate this transformation [73]. The literature suggests that CHWs may be helpful in achieving specific patient and population health goals in underserved communities with high rates of chronic disease and complex health needs. The integration of CHWs into a comprehensive care model shows some promise for improving health outcomes, particularly for interventions targeting vulnerable populations, by addressing health disparities concurrently with chronic disease prevention and management strategies. Although existing research remains limited, some evidence also suggests that using CHWs to provide health care services can be cost-effective. In addition, the patient navigation services that CHWs provide may make integration of these workers into care teams an appealing strategy for organizations and practices. Although the literature is promising overall, the variable and context-dependent outcomes seen in the U.S. to date make it difficult currently to justify broad, national policies to deploy CHWs into the health workforce and provide reimbursement for all of their services. Additional research is still needed to test and identify the most effective and economical ways that CHWs can be deployed, particularly where existing evidence is lacking or contradictory. Initiatives funded through the CMS Innovation Center may provide prototypic models for how to successfully deploy CHWs to achieve national public health aims. As promising practices for CHW training and deployment are further identified, optimal approaches for integrating CHWs into the national health care workforce should become more evident, and CHWs may take on a more clearly defined role in health care delivery reform efforts.

Appendix A: CDC Assessment of Policy Impact Potential for CHW Interventions

Category	Potential for Policy Impact*	Conclusions Drawn
Use in Chronic Disease Management	Best potential	Evidence supports that CHWs largely provide chronic disease care services, consistent with the IOM recommendation that CHWs be used in the prevention and control of chronic diseases [74].
Health-related outcomes	Best potential	CHW interventions improve access to and use of care, patients' understanding of their condition and self-management, health status, and some social outcomes.
Settings for interventions	Best potential	Evidence supports the use of CHWs in urban, rural, clinical, community, emergency department, and regional settings.
Populations served	Best potential	Outcomes often best achieved for groups historically experiencing health disparities: low income; uninsured; and racial and ethnic groups (African American, Asian, Filipino, Bangladeshi, Vietnamese, and Hispanic populations).
Cost and cost-effectiveness	Best potential	Two studies found that interventions were low cost, one demonstrated cost-effectiveness (e.g., gains in Quality Adjusted Life Years compared with usual care) and two found Medicaid cost savings.
Integration in Team-Based Care	Best potential	A mix of evidence by credible sources, including the IOM and peer-reviewed journals, supported inclusion of CHWs in multidisciplinary health care teams by demonstrating improved health-related outcomes, particularly in clinic settings and for groups experiencing health disparities (low-income, uninsured, African American, Filipino, and Hispanic populations). Lower level evidence suggested this is a low-cost approach.
Supervision by a health care provider	Best potential	CHWs practicing under provider supervision (nurse practitioner or physician) resulted in cost savings and improvement in some health, patient self-management, chronic disease, and social outcomes—especially in community-based settings, an emergency department, and for patient groups with health disparities (low-income, uninsured, African American populations). However, supervision requirements could limit the benefit of Medicaid reimbursement for CHW interventions.
Training and Certification	Best potential	Some support from practice/theory and from peer-reviewed literature suggested that standardized core competency curricula and certification for CHWs, such as the various models at the state level, could cost-effectively improve chronic disease outcomes and promote a common base of professional knowledge among CHWs. However, other evidence suggested that this approach could limit CHW adaptability and potential to assist diverse populations.
Reimbursement by Medicaid	Best potential	Evidence suggested improvements in health and health equity-related outcomes when Medicaid reimbursed for CHW services, and improved health care access and reduced resource utilization and costs for high-level health care consumers in a regional Medicaid managed care intervention (New Mexico).
Scope of Practice	Promising	Three studies supported using certification standards for providing specialty health care services (e.g., for the treatment of specific diseases such as hypertension), showing that these improved health-related outcomes. These studies were run in various settings and focused on patient groups with health disparities (low-income and African American populations).

Category	Potential for Policy Impact*	Conclusions Drawn
		One intervention resulted in a large cost savings.
Reimbursement by Private Insurance	Emerging	Evidence suggested that some private insurers cover and reimburse CHW services, which could help support CHW interventions, although little evidence suggested this improved health-related outcomes.
Educational Campaigns to Support Integration	Emerging	Limited evidence from practice and theory, largely by nonprofit and government organizations, supported use of educational campaigns to promote integration of CHWs and increase acceptance into the health care system.
Grants to Support Integration	Emerging	Limited evidence suggested grants and other financial incentives to promote the CHW workforce and support its development could lead to enhanced CHW interventions, broadening of their reach, and improving health outcomes.

*The CDC assessed strength of the evidence base by using the Quality and Impact of Component (QuIC) Evidence Assessment method [75], which categorizes research and practice sources of both empirical and non-empirical support for a policy area on a continuum of Emerging, Promising Impact, Promising Quality, and Best to suggest potential impact.

Appendix B: Opportunities for CHW Service Reimbursement through Medicaid

Mechanism	Approach	State Example
Essential Health Benefits – Preventive Services Rule	In January 2014, CMS issued a final rule (CMS-2334-F) [76, 77] giving states a new option to provide Medicaid reimbursement for preventive services recommended by, rather than provided directly by, a physician or other licensed practitioner. Hence, direct patient services can be furnished at the recommendation of a licensed provider by another health worker, such as a CHW, who may or may not be formally licensed by the state. The preventive benefit at 42 CFR 440.130(c) requires providers to furnish direct medical care for the express purpose of diagnosing, treating or preventing illness, injury or other impairments to an individual's physical or mental health, and that is directed at the patient rather than at the patient's environment.	States electing this option must submit a State Plan Amendment (SPA) to the Center for Medicaid and CHIP Services (CMCS) specifying what direct medical patient services they propose to cover; what providers will furnish these services; the required education/training, credentialing, and licensure of these providers; and the reimbursement methodology. As of November 2, 2015, no state had submitted an SPA to reimburse for CHW services [78].
Direct Reimbursement Arrangements	Although some private insurance policies may directly reimburse for CHW services, this is uncommon in Medicaid. However, state Medicaid offices may opt to develop a direct reimbursement arrangement with a provider, community, or tribal organization, making a CHW a billable provider [79]. Such arrangements specify allowable reimbursement rates as well as the	The Minnesota legislature passed a law in 2007 allowing Medicaid reimbursement for CHW health education services provided under supervision of a Medicaid-approved physician or advanced practice nurse [80, 81]. CHWs must first earn a certificate from an accredited post-secondary school offering the state-approved curriculum. CMCS

Appendix B: (Continued)

Mechanism	Approach	State Example
	education, training, and certification requirements for providers.	approved an SPA authorizing these payments. Minnesota later expanded supervisory requirements to include government public health nurses and dentists. CMCS approved both changes.
Capitation	A state Medicaid office, through a Medicaid Managed Care Organization (MCO), may pay a capitated (per-member/per-month) amount to a health plan employing CHWs directly, or a contracted amount to a community-based organization employing CHWs, who in turn pay the CHWs' salaries so long as this is in accordance with the contract and both federal and state regulations [82]. Federal regulations don't allow CMS to recognize CHWs as a provider qualifying for direct service reimbursement, but also don't prohibit CHW employment [83].	Medicaid Managed Care serves up to 70 percent of all Medicaid enrollees nationally and aims to manage costs, utilization, and quality by delivering health services through contracted arrangements.84 Health Plus, a large MCO in New York City, utilizes CHWs to deliver targeted outreach, provide community-based education, perform health risk assessments, make referrals to case managers, schedule/facilitate appointments (e.g., prenatal and well-child visits), assist in targeted clinical interventions, and offer home visits and emergency department follow-up [85, 86].
Waivers and Other Statutory Authorities	Under Section 1115 of the Social Security Act, the HHS Secretary can approve a state Medicaid program pilot for an innovative, budget-neutral demonstration project promoting CMCS objectives but providing services not traditionally covered, expanding coverage eligibility, or able to improve care or lower costs [87]. Other Medicaid waiver options and statutory authorities include Delivery System Reform Incentive Payment (DSRIP) waivers [88], Section 1915(b) Managed Care Waivers, Section1915(c) Home- and Community-Based Services Waivers [89], the Enhanced Prenatal Benefit (42 CFR §440.250), Targeted Case Management (42 CFR §440.169 and 42 CFR §441.18) [90], and Section 1945 of the Affordable Care Act (Health Home State Plan Option) [91].	Through a Section 1115 waiver initially approved by CMCS in 1999 and after three years of already functioning through state program funding, California expanded Medicaid services statewide through the Family PACT (Planning, Access, Care and Treatment) Program. Though this program, CHWs provide family planning services to 1.8 million low-income Californians today [92, 93].
State Support of Administrative Costs	Since 2005 CMCS has matched 50-75 percent of state Medicaid administrative expenses related to staffing/operating state Medicaid offices and clinics to better achieve cost control, improve information technology infrastructure, and provide interpreter, outreach, and coordination services – some activities may include using CHWs [94].	The Blue Ridge Area Health Education Center (AHEC) in Virginia's Shenandoah Valley employs bilingual CHWs as health care interpreters, with up to 40 percent of administrative costs (i.e., worker salaries but not interpreter costs) reimbursable by state Medicaid. Their Promotores de Salud program has trained over 200 Spanish-speaking lay health promoters to work with members of the local community [95, 96].

APPENDIX C: CMS INNOVATION CENTER – STATE INNOVATION MODEL TEST AWARDS

State Innovation Model Test Awards: Round One (6 states: AR, ME, MA, MN, OR, VT) Over $250 million in Model Test awards is supporting six states to implement their State Health Care Innovation Plans: proposals that describe a state's strategy to use all of the levers available to it to transform its health care delivery system through multi-payer payment reform and other state-led initiatives. *Source: http://innovation.cms.gov/initiatives/State-Innovations-Model-Testing/index.html*	
SIM state	CHW component of demonstration project
Arkansas	Arkansas has a health workforce goal of defining requirements for care coordinators, including the number and geographic distribution, skills and training curricula. The state is focusing on five core characteristics of successful population-based care, including team-based care coordination. Multi-disciplinary teams, including primary care providers, care coordinators, and support services providers, will collaborate to improve care planning, diagnosis, treatment, patient coaching to ensure treatment adherence, and management through transitions of care. Teams will extend their reach beyond the walls of the hospital or physician's office to include pharmacists, social workers, and others.
Maine	Maine will pilot a community health worker (CHW) model designed to leverage existing community connections to address the population health needs of underserved populations.
Massachusetts	Massachusetts will use a Comprehensive Primary Care Payment (CPCP) model that would give practices added flexibility to provide the right kind of care at the right time and in the right setting. This payment model may support expanding the care team, offering phone and email consultations, allowing group appointments, targeting appointment length to patient complexity, leveraging community health workers, etc., while allowing a range of primary care practice types and sizes to participate and to operationalize behavioral health integration.
Minnesota	Minnesota will be piloting the concept of Accountable Communities for Health (ACHs) – and will implement population-based prevention strategies and integrate care across the spectrum of health care and social services through development of multi-disciplinary teams, which may include emerging professions such as community health workers, community paramedics, and dental therapists. ACHs will empower and involve citizens to set measurable and measured community-based goals for improved population health, health care and cost management, and take specific steps to achieve
Oregon	Oregon's Coordinated Care Model is expressly intended to change how health care services are delivered with a strong focus on primary and preventive care and more effective care management, especially across transitions of care, and on integration of physical and behavioral health services, as well as better coordination with non-coordinated care organization services such as long-term support services and intellectually and developmentally disabled services. Patient-centered primary care homes; proactive, collaborative care planning; ongoing community health needs assessments; evidence-based practices; health information technology and broader use of nontraditional health care workers (e.g., community health workers, peer wellness specialists) are key strategies that Oregon's model are expected to use to improve health and reduce health disparities. The state plans to establish systems for training certifying non-traditional health workers, and plans to certify 300 new community health workers by December 2015.

Appendix C: (Continued)

State Innovation Model Test Awards: Round One (6 states: AR, ME, MA, MN, OR, VT) Over $250 million in Model Test awards is supporting six states to implement their State Health Care Innovation Plans: proposals that describe a state's strategy to use all of the levers available to it to transform its health care delivery system through multi-payer payment reform and other state-led initiatives. *Source: http://innovation.cms.gov/initiatives/State-Innovations-Model-Testing/index.html*	
Vermont	Vermont has developed and implemented the nationally recognized multi-payer Blueprint for Health, which is supported in part by the Center for Medicare and Medicaid Innovation's Multi-payer Advanced Primary Care Practice (MPAPCP) demonstration project. This includes extended community health teams, including the Medicaid care coordinators that are part of the Vermont Chronic Care Initiative, Support and Services at Home (SASH). These initiatives will continue to be advanced to reach specific state-defined care coordination targets.
State Innovation Model Test Awards: Round Two (11 states: CO, CT, DE, ID, IA, MI, NY, RI, OH, TN, WA) The State Innovation Models Initiative Model Test Awards will provide financial and technical support over a four-year period for states to test and evaluate multi-payer health system transformation models. States must produce and implement a detailed and fully developed proposal capable of creating state-wide health transformation for the majority of care within the state. Source: http://innovation.cms.gov/initiatives/State-Innovations-Model-Testing-Round-Two/index.html	
SIM state	CHW component of demonstration project
Colorado	Colorado is developing standard, consensus-based criteria for community health workers and patient navigators that will support both professionals and training programs. The Colorado Department of Public Health and Environment will require funds to support initiatives and infrastructure related to population health. These funds will cover personnel who will be tasked with overseeing the establishment of a state certification program for community health workers and patient navigators.
Connecticut	Connecticut plans to develop training and certification standards for Community Health Workers to help ensure that CHWs with common core competencies become an integral part of the health care workforce.
Delaware	Delaware will complement the care delivery and payment innovations with a new approach to population health that puts Delaware on a path to be one of the top five healthiest states in the nation. The core innovation is the "Healthy Neighborhoods" model, which integrates communities with their local care delivery systems, and better connects community resources with each other. Integration will be achieved through dedicated staff and a Neighborhood Council of community organizations, employers, and providers (including care coordinators and community health workers who lead care coordination in the community and across clinical settings). These connections will be reinforced with a set of common goals to ensure providers and community organizations share a focus on health, wellness, prevention, and primary care.
Idaho	Idaho's model maximizes the use of the existing health care workforce by adopting a team-based model of care that allows each practitioner to practice at the top of their licensure. Using this approach, PCMHs will be led by physicians, nurse practitioners, or physician assistants under the supervision of a physician. Some Idaho communities are so severely under-resourced that they are unable to provide team-based care within the primary care setting. In these underserved areas, two practitioner types — community health workers (CHWs) and community health emergency medical services (EMS) personnel — will be developed and advanced as key components of PCMH team-based care. Idaho's unique PCMHs will be "virtual PCMHs," as the team working together to provide coordinated primary care will be staffed across multiple agencies in the community or region.

State Innovation Model Test Awards: Round One (6 states: AR, ME, MA, MN, OR, VT) Over $250 million in Model Test awards is supporting six states to implement their State Health Care Innovation Plans: proposals that describe a state's strategy to use all of the levers available to it to transform its health care delivery system through multi-payer payment reform and other state-led initiatives. *Source: http://innovation.cms.gov/initiatives/State-Innovations-Model-Testing/index.html*	
Iowa	In Iowa, local public health agencies will provide resources and collaborate with the delivery system through a community health worker/care coordination model. Iowa proposes to "leverage and spread existing community transformation initiatives focused on the social determinants of health," which will include the utilization of CHWs to increase access to care and to improve care coordination. Community Care Teams will act as a platform to connect the delivery system to resources available in the community and mitigate access to care challenges resulting from medical provider shortages. Teams will include social workers, pharmacists, community health workers, nurses, and others.
Michigan	A Michigan advisory committee, including State innovation leadership, assembled in 2013 to conduct a systematic review of Michigan's Public Health Code. A primary objective of updating the Code is to verify that health care professionals practice at the top of their training and licensure, and to review the overall licensing scheme for emerging health professions while being attentive to the goal of avoiding unnecessary regulation. A policy objective is to incorporate non-traditional professions, such as Community Health Workers, into service coordination while also supporting standards for the training and skill sets of these occupational groups so that their outcomes can be measured.
New York	New York's Advanced Primary Care model will be structured to support integrated delivery systems that link with NY's model health home program and with community-based providers that support health through services such as housing, transportation and employment.
Ohio	Ohio currently participates in Home and Community Based Services waiver programs to promote community based care. Specific waivers focus on the aged, individuals with disabilities, and those with developmental disabilities. These segments are among the most in need of specialized care coordination. Ohio will tailor PCMH and episode-based payments design to transform care for these populations, coordinating model design with existing programs where appropriate. Ohio will align incentives, loans, and loan repayment policies to encourage primary care and PCMH participation and also align workforce priorities. For example, licensure boards in eligible disciplines provide matching funds for the State Loan Repayment Program grant in order to support additional primary team members. These disciplines include physician assistants, nurse practitioners, certified nurse midwives, psychiatric nurse specialists, health service psychologists, licensed professional counselors, licensed clinical social workers, marriage and family therapists and registered dental hygienists, pharmacists, and community health workers.
Rhode Island	Rhode Island's Community Health Worker definition is unclear and awareness of their existence and function is low among providers. The state plans to develop uniform credentials and license requirements for CHWs, integrate services within the PCMH model, include CHWs in provider directories, ensure awareness around CHWs among care teams, develop a clear career path and opportunities for people with this credential, and create a pool of workers to support the expansion of value-based care.
Tennessee	In Tennessee, practices will promote better population health by shifting the focus of care towards prevention, health maintenance, and proactive management of chronic
	conditions. Patient Centered Medical Homes (PCMHs) will reward providers for addressing the social and behavioral determinants of health such as discussing environmental asthma triggers with parents, connecting tobacco users to the Tennessee Tobacco Quitline, and connecting patients to community social services. CHWs are not directly referred to in the state's innovation plan.

Appendix C: (Continued)

State Innovation Model Test Awards: Round One (6 states: AR, ME, MA, MN, OR, VT) Over $250 million in Model Test awards is supporting six states to implement their State Health Care Innovation Plans: proposals that describe a state's strategy to use all of the levers available to it to transform its health care delivery system through multi-payer payment reform and other state-led initiatives. *Source: http://innovation.cms.gov/initiatives/State-Innovations-Model-Testing/index.html*	
Washington	Building on Washington's broad scope and authority for its workforce, the state's innovation project will specifically focus on non-traditional workforce growth for community health workers including peer support specialists. Over the duration of the project, regulatory and legislative action also will be pursued to normalize and expand the reach of tele-medicine into health professional shortage areas. Finally, real-time, rapid assessment and dissemination of key health care employer and labor projections will inform workforce supply planning.

APPENDIX D: CMS INNOVATION CENTER – HEALTH CARE INNOVATION AWARDS

Health Care Innovation Awards Round One: Awarded Projects The CMS Innovation Center announced the first batch of awardees for the Health Care Innovation Awards on May 8, 2012 and the second (final) batch on June 15, 2012. These organizations will implement projects that aim to deliver better health, improved care, and lower costs to people enrolled in Medicare, Medicaid, and the Children's Health Insurance Program (CHIP), particularly those with the highest health care needs. Funding for these projects is for three years. The proposed/estimated 3 Year Savings should be viewed with caution as this is based on award recipients' initial applications, and the actual savings realized from finalized projects has not yet been determined. *Source: http://innovation.cms.gov/initiatives/Health-Care-Innovation-Awards/Project-Profiles.html*	
Grant recipient	CHW component of project
BEN ARCHER HEALTH CENTER Project Title: "A home visitation program for rural populations in Northern Dona Ana County, New Mexico" Geographic Reach: New Mexico Funding Amount: $1,270,845 Proposed/Estimated 3-Year Savings: $6,352,888	Using nurse health educators and community health workers to bridge the gap between patients and medical providers, aid patient navigation of the health care system, and offer services including case management, medication management, chronic disease management, preventive care, home safety assessments, and health education, thereby preventing the onset and progression of diseases and reducing complications.
CHILDREN'S HOSPITAL AND HEALTH SYSTEM, INC. Project Title: "CCHP Advanced Wrap Network" Geographic Reach: Wisconsin Funding Amount: $2,796,255	Children's Hospital and Health System received an award to create Care Links, which will support members of Children's Community Health Plan (CCHP), the system's Medicaid HMO in Southeast Wisconsin, as they navigate the health care system. Care Links will allow community health navigators to educate and empower health plan members to

Health Care Innovation Awards Round One: Awarded Projects The CMS Innovation Center announced the first batch of awardees for the Health Care Innovation Awards on May 8, 2012 and the second (final) batch on June 15, 2012. These organizations will implement projects that aim to deliver better health, improved care, and lower costs to people enrolled in Medicare, Medicaid, and the Children's Health Insurance Program (CHIP), particularly those with the highest health care needs. Funding for these projects is for three years. The proposed/estimated 3 Year Savings should be viewed with caution as this is based on award recipients' initial applications, and the actual savings realized from finalized projects has not yet been determined. *Source: http://innovation.cms.gov/initiatives/Health-Care-Innovation-Awards/Project-Profiles.html*	
Estimated 3-Year Savings: $2,851,266	navigate the health care system, connect with a primary care doctor and receive preventive care and appropriate screenings. Community health navigators will offer services to individuals and families who have had two ER visits within six months. A nurse navigator will work with health plan members diagnosed with asthma who have had one ER or one inpatient stay related to asthma. Both the community navigators and the nurse navigator will reinforce the availability of urgent care and CCHP's 24/7 nurse advice line. The goal of Care Links is to reduce avoidable ER visits, improve health outcomes (specific HEDIS measures) and reduce cost. Over the three year period, Children's Hospital and Health System will create nine jobs, including a program manager, community health navigators and nurse navigators.
COOPER UNIVERSITY HOSPITAL Project Title: N/A Geographic Reach: New Jersey Funding Amount: $2,788,457 Estimated 3-Year Savings: $6.2 million	Will train an estimated 22 health care workers, while creating an estimated 16 new jobs. These workers will include non-clinical staff, like AmeriCorps volunteers and community health workers, who will serve as part of the multidisciplinary teams to support care coordination activities.
DUKE UNIVERSITY/SOUTH EAST DIABETES INITIATIVE Project Title: From clinic to community: achieving health equity in the southern United States Funding Amount: $9,773,499 Estimated 3 Year Savings: $20.8M	Uses risk algorithms (social and clinical) and geospatial software to target "hot spot" communities within 4 counties in NC, MS, and WV in need of intensive Type 2 Diabetes care; delivers enhanced, coordinated, patient-centered team care (including home visits) to High risk, telephonic interventions to Medium and community based programs to Low risk groups) provided by local care teams, including extensive use of CHWs.
EAU CLAIRE COOPERATIVE HEALTH CENTERS, INC. Project Title: "Healthy Columbia: recruiting, training, organizing, deploying, and supporting community health teams in low income area of Columbia, South Carolina" Geographic Reach: South Carolina	Eau Claire Cooperative Health Centers, Inc., in partnership with the Select Health and BlueChoice Medicaid Managed Care Organizations, is receiving an award for a project aimed at improving health outcomes for populations in underserved, low-income areas of Columbia, South Carolina. Eau Claire will use health care teams of nurse practitioners, registered nurses, and community health workers affiliated with a Federally Qualified Health Center to provide patient education, home visits, and care coordination, leading to reduced use of high cost health care services, including

Appendix D: (Continued)

Health Care Innovation Awards Round One: Awarded Projects The CMS Innovation Center announced the first batch of awardees for the Health Care Innovation Awards on May 8, 2012 and the second (final) batch on June 15, 2012. These organizations will implement projects that aim to deliver better health, improved care, and lower costs to people enrolled in Medicare, Medicaid, and the Children's Health Insurance Program (CHIP), particularly those with the highest health care needs. Funding for these projects is for three years. The proposed/estimated 3 Year Savings should be viewed with caution as this is based on award recipients' initial applications, and the actual savings realized from finalized projects has not yet been determined. *Source: http://innovation.cms.gov/initiatives/Health-Care-Innovation-Awards/Project-Profiles.html*	
Funding Amount: $2,330,000 Estimated 3-Year Savings: $14,817,600	emergency room visits and hospitalizations, improved self-management for patients with chronic conditions, a decrease in low birth weight infant care, and improved health outcomes in general. Payers have agreed to reimburse a portion of cost savings. Over a three-year period, Eau Claire Cooperative Health Centers will create an estimated 22 health care-related jobs, including positions for peer health workers, registered nurses, Nurse Practitioners, and a project director.
FINITY COMMUNICATIONS, INC. Project Title: "EveryBODY Get Healthy" Geographic Reach: Pennsylvania Funding Amount: $4,967,962 Estimated 3-Year Savings: $8.7 million	The Finity Communications, Inc. model is designed to improve health care for over 120,000 high-need Medicaid beneficiaries in the Greater Philadelphia area. The innovation uses health analytics technology to track risk criteria and update integrated health profiles, and to deploy targeted alerts, outreach, wellness, and support services in a closed-loop environment that evolves with successful behavioral change. The innovation includes providing Peer Mentors to support ongoing engagement and healthy behavioral change. This integrated approach to health care is expected to reduce the gaps in care and lead to improved health care, better health, and reduced costs for individuals with diabetes, heart disease, hypertension, asthma, and high-risk pregnancy.
FIRSTVITALS HEALTH AND WELLNESS INC. Project Title: Improving the health and care of low-income diabetics at reduced costs 3 Year Funding Amount: $3,999,713 Estimated 3 Year Savings: $4,829,955	Partnering with AlohaCare, a large health plan in Hawaii with 70,000 Medicaid members, FirstVitals reaches out and engaging hard to reach patients with diabetes who already have neuropathy (determined through a device known as a DPN-Check,) which indicates poor control. Uses technology, such as a wireless glucometer to monitor patients with diabetes, tablets to keep them informed and socially networked and deploys Integrated Care Coordinators (similar to CHWs) to improve diabetes management for target population.
FOUNDATION FOR CALIFORNIA COMMUNITY COLLEGES Project Title: "Transitions clinic network: linking high-risk Medicaid patients from prison to community primary care"	Targeting eleven community health centers (in six states, the District of Columbia, and Puerto Rico), and working with the Department of Corrections to identify patients with chronic medical conditions prior to release. Will use community health workers trained by the City College of San Francisco to help these individuals navigate the health care system,

Health Care Innovation Awards Round One: Awarded Projects The CMS Innovation Center announced the first batch of awardees for the Health Care Innovation Awards on May 8, 2012 and the second (final) batch on June 15, 2012. These organizations will implement projects that aim to deliver better health, improved care, and lower costs to people enrolled in Medicare, Medicaid, and the Children's Health Insurance Program (CHIP), particularly those with the highest health care needs. Funding for these projects is for three years. The proposed/estimated 3 Year Savings should be viewed with caution as this is based on award recipients' initial applications, and the actual savings realized from finalized projects has not yet been determined. *Source: http://innovation.cms.gov/initiatives/Health-Care-Innovation-Awards/Project-Profiles.html*	
Geographic Reach: Alabama, California, Connecticut, District of Columbia, Maryland, Massachusetts, New York, Puerto Rico Funding Amount: $6,852,153 Estimated 3-Year Savings: $8,115,855	find primary care and other medical and social services, and coach them in chronic disease management. The outcomes will include reduced reliance on emergency room care, fewer hospital admissions, and lower cost, with improved patient health and better access to appropriate care.
HEALTH RESOURCES IN ACTION Project Title: "New England asthma innovations collaborative" Geographic Reach: Connecticut, Massachusetts, Rhode Island, Vermont Funding Amount: $4,040,657 Estimated 3-Year Savings: $4.1 million	Rapid service delivery expansion for over 1300 high-risk children with asthma in Connecticut, Rhode Island, Massachusetts, and Vermont. NEAIC employs the following components of care: 1) Asthma self-management education 2) Home environmental assessment with the provision of minor-to-moderate environmental intervention supplies to reduce asthma triggers; and 3) Use of non-physician providers shown to be cost-effective deliverers of this level of care, particularly community health workers (CHWs) and certified asthma educators (AE-Cs).
JOHNS HOPKINS UNIVERSITY Project Title: "Johns Hopkins Community Health Partnership (J-CHiP)" Geographic Reach: Maryland Funding Amount: $19,920,338 Estimated 3-Year Savings: $52,600,000	Over a three-year period, will train and hire more than 75 new health care workers, including nurse educators, nurse transition guides, case managers, community health workers, and health behavior specialists (and will retrain care coordinators, patient access line case managers, clinical pharmacy specialists, community health workers, and physicians already on staff) to increase access to services for high-risk adults in East Baltimore, MD – especially those with chronic illness, mental illness, and/or substance abuse conditions. The intervention improves care coordination across the continuum and comprises early risk screening, interdisciplinary care planning, enhanced medication management, patient/family education, provider communication, post-discharge support and home care services, including self-management coaching, and improved access to primary care.
JOSLIN DIABETES CENTER, INC.	Expands a diabetes education program, known as "On the Road" delivered by Community Health

Appendix D: (Continued)

Health Care Innovation Awards Round One: Awarded Projects The CMS Innovation Center announced the first batch of awardees for the Health Care Innovation Awards on May 8, 2012 and the second (final) batch on June 15, 2012. These organizations will implement projects that aim to deliver better health, improved care, and lower costs to people enrolled in Medicare, Medicaid, and the Children's Health Insurance Program (CHIP), particularly those with the highest health care needs. Funding for these projects is for three years. The proposed/estimated 3 Year Savings should be viewed with caution as this is based on award recipients' initial applications, and the actual savings realized from finalized projects has not yet been determined. *Source: http://innovation.cms.gov/initiatives/Health-Care-Innovation-Awards/Project-Profiles.html*	
Project Title: "Pathways to better health through a new health care workforce and community" Geographic Reach: District of Columbia, New Mexico, Pennsylvania Funding Amount: $4,967,276 Estimated 3-Year Savings: $7.4 million	Advocates (similar to CHWs) and health educators, working with Cooperative Extension Services in PA, NM, and testing this approach with an urban population, through an inner city hospital in DC. They met their target goal of 5100 participants with diabetes, pre-diabetes or family members (primarily Medicare and Medicaid beneficiaries), with goal of preventing or better managing diabetes.
LE BONHEUR COMMUNITY HEALTH AND WELL BEING Project Title: "Le Bonheur's CHAMP Program: Changing High-risk Asthma in Memphis through Partnership" Geographic Reach: Memphis and Shelby County, Tennessee Funding Amount: $2,896,416 Estimated 3-Year Savings: $4,003,397	The Community Coordination team, comprised of two Asthma Care Coordinators and 4 Community Health Workers who are supervised by a Licensed Clinical Social Worker, provides asthma education; environmental assessment; coordination with schools and child care; and provides help with barriers to asthma management.
MICHIGAN PUBLIC HEALTH INSTITUTE Project Title: "Michigan pathways to better health" Geographic Reach: Michigan Funding Amount: $14,145,784 Estimated 3-Year Savings: $17,498,641	Implements the Pathways Innovation through the "Pathways Community Hub" and elements of the Collective Impact models (e.g., backbone organizations;) integrating community health workers (CHWs) into primary care teams in MI, (Ingham, Saginaw and Muskegon Counties) by assessing at risk adults with 2 or more chronic diseases; designing a value based payment model for CHWs. CHWs coach patients on chronic disease self-management and connect at-risk populations with care and support services that address social determinants of health, such as primary care, housing, food, and transportation, as well as their clinical and mental health needs.
THE NATIONAL HEALTH CARE FOR THE HOMELESS COUNCIL Project Title: "Community health workers and HCH: a partnership to promote primary care" Geographic Reach: California, Illinois, Massachusetts, Nebraska, New Hampshire, North Carolina, Ohio, Texas Funding Amount: $2,681,877 Estimated 3-Year Savings: $1.5 million	Working with twelve communities across various regions in the U.S. to reduce the number of emergency department visits and lack of primary care services for over 500 homeless individuals. The intervention integrates community health workers into Federally Qualified Health Centers to conduct outreach and case coordination for transitioning this population from the emergency department to a health center, thus reducing unnecessary emergency department visits and improving quality of care for the homeless population.

Health Care Innovation Awards Round One: Awarded Projects The CMS Innovation Center announced the first batch of awardees for the Health Care Innovation Awards on May 8, 2012 and the second (final) batch on June 15, 2012. These organizations will implement projects that aim to deliver better health, improved care, and lower costs to people enrolled in Medicare, Medicaid, and the Children's Health Insurance Program (CHIP), particularly those with the highest health care needs. Funding for these projects is for three years. The proposed/estimated 3 Year Savings should be viewed with caution as this is based on award recipients' initial applications, and the actual savings realized from finalized projects has not yet been determined. *Source: http://innovation.cms.gov/initiatives/Health-Care-Innovation-Awards/Project-Profiles.html*	
NEMOURS ALFRED I. DUPONT HOSPITAL FOR CHILDREN Project Title: "Optimizing health outcomes for children with asthma in Delaware" Geographic Reach: Delaware Funding Amount: $3,697,300 Estimated 3-Year Savings: $4,743,184	The intervention will increase coordination of services by integrating care with community support services and local government initiatives to provide healthier environments for children with asthma in schools, child care centers, and housing, and by deploying community health workers to serve as patient navigators and provide case management services to families with high needs.
RUTGERS, THE STATE UNIVERSITY OF NEW JERSEY (THE CENTER FOR STATE HEALTH POLICY) Project Title: "Sustainable high-utilization team model" Geographic Reach: California, Colorado, Missouri, Pennsylvania Funding Amount: $14,347,808 Estimated 3-Year Savings: $67,719,052	Will expand and test a team-based care management strategy for high-cost, high-need, low-income populations served by safety-net provider organizations in Allentown, PA, Aurora, CO, Kansas City, MO, and San Diego, CA. The project will use integrated care management teams (including nurses, social workers, and community health workers) to provide clients with patient-centered support that addresses both health care needs and the underlying determinants of health. Teams will assist patients in managing chronic illness, including filling prescriptions and coordinating appropriate specialty care, in addition to addressing social service needs such as identifying stable housing, applying for health coverage or disability benefits and facilitating transportation arrangements.
UNIVERSITY EMERGENCY MEDICAL SERVICES Project Title: "Better health through social and health care linkages beyond the emergency department" Geographic Reach: New York Funding Amount: $2,570,749	Is deploying community health workers to work with frequent emergency department (ED) utilizers and meaningfully link them to primary care, social and health services, education, and provide health coaching. The program targets 2,300 Medicare and Medicaid beneficiaries who have had two or more emergency department visits over 12 months in urban Buffalo, New York.
Estimated 3-Year Savings: $6.1 million	
UNIVERSITY OF CHICAGO Project Title: "CommunityRx system: linking patients and community-based service" Geographic Reach: Illinois Funding Amount: $5,862,027 Estimated 3-Year Savings: $6.4 million	The University of Chicago Urban Health Initiative in partnership with Chicago Health Information Technology Regional Extension Center (CHITREC) and the Alliance of Chicago Community Health Services received an award to develop the CommunityRx system, a continuously updated electronic database of community health resources that will be linked to the Electronic Health Records of local safety net providers. In real time, the system will process patient data and print out a "HealtheRx" for the patient, including

Appendix D: (Continued)

Health Care Innovation Awards Round One: Awarded Projects The CMS Innovation Center announced the first batch of awardees for the Health Care Innovation Awards on May 8, 2012 and the second (final) batch on June 15, 2012. These organizations will implement projects that aim to deliver better health, improved care, and lower costs to people enrolled in Medicare, Medicaid, and the Children's Health Insurance Program (CHIP), particularly those with the highest health care needs. Funding for these projects is for three years. The proposed/estimated 3 Year Savings should be viewed with caution as this is based on award recipients' initial applications, and the actual savings realized from finalized projects has not yet been determined. *Source: http://innovation.cms.gov/initiatives/Health-Care-Innovation-Awards/Project-Profiles.html*	
	referrals to community resources relevant to the patient's condition and status. Aggregated data on patient diagnoses and referrals will be used to generate CommunityRx reports for community-based service providers to use to inform programming. The program will serve over 200,000 patients on the South Side of Chicago most of whom are Medicare, Medicaid and CHIP beneficiaries. The CommunityRx system will train and create new jobs for a combined total of over 200 individuals from this high-poverty, diverse community. This includes high school youth who will collect data on community health resources as part of the Urban Health Initiative's MAPSCorps program. It will also include the creation of a new type of health worker, Community Health Information Experts (CHIEs), who will assist patients in using the HealtheRx and engage community-based service providers in meaningful use of the CommunityRx reports. The CommunityRx builds on infrastructure supported by ARRA funding from the National Institute on Aging. Anticipated outcomes include better population health, better use of appropriate services, increased compliance with care, and fewer avoidable visits to the emergency room with estimated savings of approximately $6.4 million.
UNIVERSITY OF MIAMI Project Title: "Expanded activities of school health initiative" Geographic Reach: Florida Funding Amount: $4,097,198 Estimated 3-Year Savings: $5,620,017	Goal to improve care and access to care for children in four communities in the Miami-Dade County area who have health problems that include asthma, obesity, type II diabetes, and STDs. This intervention has resulted in an expansion of services and utility of school-based health clinics, increased collaboration with other care providers, services, and school-health stakeholders, and enhanced usage and sharing of health information technology. A team-based approach is being utilized to improve care and quality of services. This approach incorporates community health workers, nursing assistants, and dental hygienists while taking advantage of telehealth opportunities. The program will lower cost through preventive and more appropriate care and increase access to care, services, and benefits.

Health Care Innovation Awards Round One: Awarded Projects The CMS Innovation Center announced the first batch of awardees for the Health Care Innovation Awards on May 8, 2012 and the second (final) batch on June 15, 2012. These organizations will implement projects that aim to deliver better health, improved care, and lower costs to people enrolled in Medicare, Medicaid, and the Children's Health Insurance Program (CHIP), particularly those with the highest health care needs. Funding for these projects is for three years. The proposed/estimated 3 Year Savings should be viewed with caution as this is based on award recipients' initial applications, and the actual savings realized from finalized projects has not yet been determined. *Source: http://innovation.cms.gov/initiatives/Health-Care-Innovation-Awards/Project-Profiles.html*	
Health Care Innovation Awards Round Two: Awarded Projects The CMS Innovation Center announced the first batch of prospective recipients for the Health Care Innovation Awards Round Two on May 22, 2014 and the second batch on July 9, 2014. The cumulative 39 awards are being implemented in 27 states and the District of Columbia spanning a wide range of patient populations, from children to the elderly, across the care continuum. The Health Care Innovation Awards Round Two are funding up to $1 billion in awards and evaluation to applicants across the country that test new payment and service delivery models that will deliver better care and lower costs for Medicare, Medicaid, and/or CHIP enrollees. Source: http://innovation.cms.gov/initiatives/Health-Care-Innovation-Awards/Round-2.html	
Grant recipient	CHW component of project
CHILDREN'S HOME SOCIETY OF FLORIDA Project Title: Improving child well-being through integrating care in a community school setting Geographic Reach: Florida Estimated Funding Amount: $2,078,295	Will implement a medical home for students, families, teachers and the community at the Wellness Cottage at Evans High School, which aims to reduce Emergency Department and inpatient utilization, increase sexually transmitted disease awareness, and address food insecurities and traumatic stress. Four community partners including Children's Home Society of Florida (child welfare/behavioral health), the University of Central Florida, Orange County Public Schools and Central Florida Family Health Center will operate the Wellness Cottage, a hub for health, social, behavioral health, parental support, and after-school activities. The Central Florida Family Health
	Center will provide onsite primary care. Health risk assessments will inform health promotion activities. Student health ambassadors will promote healthy lifestyles. Community health workers will help parents remove barriers to care. The University of Central Florida will provide social work, nursing, and medical interns. Primary Health Maintenance Organizations will facilitate access to the clinic and assist in evaluating health costs. Programs and services targeting wellness will be available in the school and community.
CLIFFORD W. BEERS GUIDANCE CLINIC, INC. Project Title: New Haven WrapAround Geographic Reach: Connecticut Estimated Funding Amount: $9,739,427	Will deliver evidence-based, culturally-appropriate integrated medical, behavioral health, and community-based services coordinated by a multidisciplinary Wraparound Team. Services include: 1) family engagement, recruitment, and education provided by trained community health workers in community-based settings; 2) multidisciplinary triage, screening, and assessment conducted by the Wraparound Team and including assessments

Appendix D: (Continued)

<table>
<tr><td colspan="2">Health Care Innovation Awards Round One: Awarded Projects
The CMS Innovation Center announced the first batch of awardees for the Health Care Innovation Awards on May 8, 2012 and the second (final) batch on June 15, 2012. These organizations will implement projects that aim to deliver better health, improved care, and lower costs to people enrolled in Medicare, Medicaid, and the Children's Health Insurance Program (CHIP), particularly those with the highest health care needs. Funding for these projects is for three years. The proposed/estimated 3 Year Savings should be viewed with caution as this is based on award recipients' initial applications, and the actual savings realized from finalized projects has not yet been determined.
Source: http://innovation.cms.gov/initiatives/Health-Care-Innovation-Awards/Project-Profiles.html</td></tr>
<tr><td></td><td>of each family's physical, behavioral, and psychosocial risks, needs, and strengths; 3) family-focused care plans developed with the family, family supports, and the Wraparound Team and used to guide care and interventions; 4) care coordination provided by a Wraparound Team and focused on coordinating the provision of appropriate care across multiple care settings, managing care transitions, reconciling and managing medications, and coordinating access to crisis support and wellness and social support services; and 5) wellness and social support services provided at the hubs and at community-based organizations to address chronic and toxic stress (e.g., smoking cessation, parenting courses, diabetes prevention, meditation). The model focuses on high-need families, addresses medical and behavioral health care needs, integrates services across multiple health care institutions, and addresses the "chronic and toxic stress" experienced by the target population families.</td></tr>
<tr><td>GEORGE WASHINGTON UNIVERSITY
Project Title: PREVENTION AT HOME: A Model for Novel use of Mobile Technologies and Integrated Care Systems to Improve HIV Prevention and Care While Lowering Cost
Geographic Reach: Washington D.C.
Estimated Funding Amount: $23,808,617</td><td>Will test a model that will utilize mobile technologies and optimize the prevention and care continuum (early detection, treatment adherence, retention in care, viral load suppression, decreased hospitalizations) for HIV+ individuals. Will bring together a consortium of stakeholders including community outreach organizations, clinical care systems, a hospital, a managed care organization, the DC Department of Health, and DC Medicaid to share integrated IT systems. Together these systems will provide Medicaid members with the ability to receive online education, the option of ordering home testing and home specimen collection for sexually transmitted infections and HIV, receive sexually transmitted infection and viral load test results, receive e-prescriptions and support linking and relinking to care. Additionally, the systems will provide community health workers (CHW) with a mobile tool to collect recruitment data, to guide counseling, testing and linkage services, and will provide CHW with a list of active patients to provide care coordination who have detectable viral load, missed clinic visits, missed medication refills, emergency room visits</td></tr>
</table>

Health Care Innovation Awards Round One: Awarded Projects

The CMS Innovation Center announced the first batch of awardees for the Health Care Innovation Awards on May 8, 2012 and the second (final) batch on June 15, 2012. These organizations will implement projects that aim to deliver better health, improved care, and lower costs to people enrolled in Medicare, Medicaid, and the Children's Health Insurance Program (CHIP), particularly those with the highest health care needs. Funding for these projects is for three years. The proposed/estimated 3 Year Savings should be viewed with caution as this is based on award recipients' initial applications, and the actual savings realized from finalized projects has not yet been determined.

Source: http://innovation.cms.gov/initiatives/Health-Care-Innovation-Awards/Project-Profiles.html

	or hospitalizations.
THE TRUSTEES OF COLUMBIA UNIVERSITY IN THE CITY OF NEW YORK Project Title: MySmileBuddy": Demonstrating the Value of Technology-assisted Non-surgical Care Management in Young Children Geographic Reach: New York Estimated Funding Amount: $3,870,446	Will test a model that uses family-level, peer-counseled, and technology-assisted behavioral risk reduction strategies, aims to divert children with early- and advanced-stage early childhood caries (ECC) from high-cost surgical dental rehabilitation (DR) to low-cost non-surgical disease management (NSDM). Together, parents and community health workers (CHWs) will use MySmileBuddy (MSB), a mobile tablet-based health technology, to plan, implement, and monitor positive oral health behaviors, including dietary control and use of fluorides, which arrest ECC's progression.

REFERENCES

[1] Patient Protection and Affordable Care Act of 2010. PL 111-148, secs. 5101, 5102, 5313, 5403, and 3509.

[2] Shah MK, Heisler M, Davis MM. Community health workers and the Patient Protection and Affordable Care Act: an opportunity for a research, advocacy, and policy agenda. J Health Care Poor Underserved. 2014 Feb; 25(1): 17-24.

[3] Bureau of Labor Statistics. Standard Occupational Classification. Community Health Workers. 2010. Acquired April 30, 2015 from: http://www.bls.gov/soc/2010/soc211094.htm.

[4] Community Health Workers. The American Public Health Association. Acquired July 13, 2015 from: https://www.apha.org/aphacommunities/member-sections/community-health-workers/.

[5] Brownstein JN, Hirsch GR, Rosenthal EL, Rush C. Community Health Workers "101" for Primary Care Providers and Other Stakeholders in Health Care Systems. J Ambulatory Care Management 2011 Jul-Sep;34(3): 210-220.

[6] American Public Health Association. Community Health Workers. Acquired June 3, 2015 from: https://www.apha.org/aphacommunities/member-sections/community-health-workers/.

[7] Lehmann U, Sanders D. Community health workers: What do we know about them? The state of the evidence on programmes, activities, costs and impact on health outcomes of using community health workers. World Health Organization. January 2007. Acquired June 3, 2015 from: http://www.who.int/hrh/documents/community_health_workers.pdf.

[8] Who Are Community Health Workers? Mass.gov. The Official Website of the Executive Office of Health and Human Services (EOHHS). Acquired June 3, 2015 from: http://www.mass.gov/eohhs/gov/departments/dph/programs/community-health/primarycare-healthaccess/healthcareworkforce-center/comm-health-wkrs/who-are-community-health-workers.html.

[9] Shah MK, Heisler M, Davis MM. Community health workers and the Patient Protection and Affordable Care Act: an opportunity for a research, advocacy, and policy agenda. J Health Care Poor Underserved. 2014 Feb; 25(1): 17-24.

[10] California Health Workforce Alliance. Taking Innovation to Scale: Community Health Workers, Promotors, and the Triple Aim. 2013. Acquired April 30, 2015 from: http://goo.gl/3XY0pZ.

[11] Viswanathan M, Kraschnewski J, Nishikawa B, Morgan LC, Thieda P, Honeycutt A, Lohr KN, Jonas D. Outcomes of Community Health Worker Interventions. Evidence Report/Technology Assessment No. 181 (Prepared by the RTI International–University of North Carolina Evidence-based Practice Center under Contract No. 290 2007 10056 I.) AHRQ Publication No. 09-E014. Rockville, MD: Agency for Healthcare Research and Quality. June 2009. Acquired April 30, 2015 from: http://www.ahrq.gov/research/findings/evidence-based-reports/comhworkevidence-report.pdf.

[12] Centers for Disease Control and Prevention. Policy Evidence Assessment Report: Community Health Worker Policy Components. Atlanta, GA: U.S. Department of Health and Human Services, Centers for Disease Control and Prevention; 2014.

Acquired April 30, 2015 from: http://www.cdc.gov/dhdsp/pubs/docs/chw_evidence_assessment_report.pdf.

[13] Centers for Disease Control and Prevention. Addressing Chronic Disease through Community Health Workers: A Policy and Systems Level Approach. Second Edition. Atlanta, GA: U.S. Department of Health and Human Services, Centers for Disease Control and Prevention. 2015. Acquired April 30, 2015 from: http://www.cdc.gov/dhdsp/docs/chw_brief.pdf.

[14] Guide to Community Preventive Services. Cardiovascular Disease Prevention and Control: Interventions Engaging Community Health Workers (abbreviated). Acquired June 1, 2015 from: http://www.thecommunity guide.org/cvd/CHW.html.

[15] Association of State and Territorial Health Officials. Building a Sustainable Community Health Worker Workforce in Massachusetts. December 2013. Acquired April 30, 2015 from: http://www.astho.org/Workforce-Committee-CHW-Presen tation-12-11-13/.

[16] Singh P, Chokshi DA. Community Health Workers—A Local Solution to a Global Problem. N Engl J Med 2013 Sep 5; 369(10):894-896.

[17] Pérez LM, Martinez J. Community Health Workers: Social Justice and Policy Advocates for Community Health and Well-Being. American Journal of Public Health. 2008;98(1): 11-14.

[18] Centers for Disease Control and Prevention. A Community Health Worker Training Resource for Preventing Heart Disease and Stroke. April 2014. Acquired November 2, 2015 at: http://www.cdc.gov/dhdsp/programs/spha/chw_sourcebook/pdfs/source book.pdf.

[19] Balcazar H, Rosenthal E, Brownstein J, Rush C, Matos S, Lorenza H. Community health workers can be a public health force for change in the United States: three actions for a new paradigm. American Journal of Public Health 2011 Dec;101(12):2199-2203.

[20] Gilkey MB, Garcia CC, Rush H. Professionalization and the experience-based expert: strengthening partnerships between health educators and community health workers. Health Promotion Practice; 2011 Mar; 12(2): 178-182.

[21] American Public Health Association. Support for Community Health Worker Leadership in Determining Workforce Standards for Training and Credentialing. Policy Number 201414; 2014. Acquired April 30, 2015 from: http://www.apha. org/policies-and-advocacy/public-healthpolicy-statements/policy-database/2015/01/28/14/15/support-for-community-health-worker-leadership.

[22] Islam N, Nadkarni SK, Zahn D, Skillman M, Kwon SC, Trinh-Shevrin C. Integrating community health workers within Patient Protection and Affordable Care Act implementation. Journal of Public Health Management Practices; 2015 Jan-Feb;21(1):42-50.

[23] California Health Workforce Alliance. Taking Innovation to Scale: Community Health Workers, Promotors, and the Triple Aim. 2013. Acquired April 30, 2015 from: http://goo.gl/3XY0pZ.

[24] Essential Hospitals Institute. Facilitators and Barriers to Providing Patient-Centered Chronic Disease Care to Patient Populations at Risk for Health and Health Care Disparities in Safety Net Settings. 2013. Acquired April 30, 2015 from:

http://www.pcori.org/assets/2014/01/PCORIFacilitators-Barriers-Providing-Patient-Centered-Chronic-Disease-Care-120613.pdf.

[25] Bodenheimer T, Chen E, Bennett HD. Confronting the growing burden of chronic disease: can the U.S. health care workforce do the job? Health Aff (Millwood). 2009 Jan-Feb;28(1): 64-74.

[26] CDC Health Disparities and Inequalities Report - United States, 2013. MMWR Supplement 2013 Nov 22; 62 Suppl 3:1-187.

[27] Centers for Disease Control and Prevention. Coronary heart disease and stroke deaths - United States, 2009. In: CDC health disparities and inequalities report - United States, 2013. MMWR 2013; 62 Suppl 3:155-158.

[28] Centers for Disease Control and Prevention. Infant deaths - United States, 2005-2008. In: CDC health disparities and inequalities report - United States, 2013. MMWR 2013;62 Suppl 3:169-172.

[29] Centers for Disease Control and Prevention. Diabetes - United States, 2006 and 2010. In: CDC health disparities and inequalities report - United States, 2013. MMWR 2013;62 Suppl 3:97-102.

[30] Joint Center for Political and Economic Studies. The economic burden of health inequalities in the United States. 2009. Washington, DC. Acquired June 1, 2015 from: http://jointcenter.org/research/fact-sheet-economic-burden-health-inequalities-united-states.

[31] US Department of Health and Human Services, Health Resources and Services Administration, Bureau of Health Professions. Community Health Worker National Workforce Study. Available at: http://bhpr.hrsa.gov/healthworkforce/reports/chwstudy2007.pdf. Accessed November 2, 2015.

[32] The Arizona Prevention Research Center of the University of Arizona. The 2014 National Community Health Worker Advocacy Survey (NCHWAS). Acquired April 30, 2015 from: http://azprc.arizona.edu/content/2014-national-community-health-worker-advocacy-survey-reports.

[33] Minnesota CHW Alliance. Education. Acquired September 24, 2015 from: http://mnchwalliance.org/explore-the-field/education-2/

[34] Willaert A. Minnesota Community Health Worker Workforce Analysis: Summary of Findings for Minneapolis and St. Paul. Mankato, Minn: Healthcare Education Industry Partnership. 2005. Acquired April 30, 2015 from: http://www.apha. org/policies-and-advocacy/public-health-policy-statements/policy-database/2014/07/09/14/19/support-for-community-health-workers-to-increase-health-access-and-to-reduce-health-inequities.

[35] The New Mexico Community Health Worker (CHW) Advisory Council (NMCHWAC). Acquired November 2, 2015 from: http://www.nmchw.org/

[36] Community Health Workers. Association of State and Territorial Health Officials. Acquired June 2, 2015 from: http://www.astho.org/community-health-workers/.

[37] Institute of Medicine. Unequal Treatment: Confronting Racial and Ethnic Disparities in Health Care (2002). Acquired June 4, 2015 from: http://www.iom.edu/Reports/2002/Unequal-Treatment-Confronting-Racial-and-Ethnic-Disparities-in-Health-Care.aspx.

[38] Miller P, Bates T, Katzen A. Community Health Worker Credentialing. State Approaches. Harvard Law School – Center for Health Law and Policy Innovation. July

16, 2014. Acquired June 4, 2015 from: http://www.chlpi.org/wp-content/ uploads/ 2014/06/CHW-CredentialingPaper.pdf.

[39] Carl H. Rush, Basics of Community Health Worker Credentialing (2012). Acquired June 4, 2015 from: http://www.chwnec.org/pdf/Basics%20of% 20Community%20 Health%20Worker%20Credentialing.pdf.

[40] Institute of Medicine. Unequal Treatment: Confronting Racial and Ethnic Disparities in Health Care (2002). Acquired June 4, 2015 from: http://www.iom.edu/Reports/ 2002/Unequal-Treatment-Confronting-Racial-and-Ethnic-Disparities-in-Health-Care.aspx.

[41] Miller P, Bates T, Katzen A. Community Health Worker Credentialing. State Approaches. Center for Health Law and Policy Innovation, Harvard Law School. July 16, 2014. Acquired June 4, 2015 from: http://www.chlpi.org/wp-content/ uploads/ 2014/06/CHW-CredentialingPaper.pdf.

[42] The Community Health Worker Core Consensus (C3) Project. Acquired November 2, 2015 from: http://chrllc.net/id12.html.

[43] Carl H. Rush, Basics of Community Health Worker Credentialing (2012). Acquired June 4, 2015 from: http://www.chwnec.org/pdf/Basics%20of%20Community% 20Health%20Worker%20Credentialing.pdf.

[44] The Arizona Prevention Research Center of the University of Arizona. The 2014 National Community Health Worker Advocacy Survey (NCHWAS). Acquired April 30, 2015 from: http://azprc.arizona.edu/content/2014-national-community-health-worker-advocacy-survey-reports.

[45] General CHR Information. Indian Health Service. Acquired October 8, 2015 from: http://www.ihs.gov/chr/index.cfm?module=history.

[46] Department of Health and Human Services. Indian Health Service. Fiscal Year 2016. Justification of Estimates for Appropriations Committees. Acquired October 8, 2015 from: http://www.ihs.gov/budgetformulation/includes/themes/newihstheme/documents/FY2016CongressionalJustification.pdf.

[47] General CHR Information. Indian Health Service. Acquired October 8, 2015 from: http://www.ihs.gov/chr/index.cfm?module=history.

[48] Personal Communication: Mose Herne – Director of Division of Planning, Evaluation and Research, Office of Public Health Support, Indian Health Service. October 27, 2015.

[49] 49 National Association of Community Health Representatives. Acquired October 8, 2015 from: http://nachr.net/index.php/about-us.html.

[50] National Association of Community Health Representatives. Survey Report. February 13, 2014. Acquired October 8, 2015 from: http://nachr.net/index.php/about-us.html.

[51] Indian Health Service HQ/OCPS/Community Health Representative. 2014. Trends in Indian Health 2014 Edition. Rockville, MD: Indian Health Services, U.S. Department of Health and Human Services.

[52] Com52 Indian Health Service HQ/OCPS/Community Health Representative. 2014. Trends in Indian Health 2014 Edition. Rockville, MD: Indian Health Services, U.S. Department of Health and Human Services.munity Health Workers, What Do We Know About Them? The state of the evidence on programs, activities, costs and impact on health outcomes of using community health workers. World Health Organization;

2007. Acquired April 30, 2015 from: http://www.who.int/hrh/documents/community health workers.pdf.

[53] Bhutta Z, Lassi Z, Pariyo G, Huicho L. Global experience of community health workers for delivery of health related Millennium Development Goals: a systematic review, country case studies, and recommendations for integration into national health systems. Geneva: World Health Organization, 2010.

[54] Community Health Workers, What Do We Know About Them? The state of the evidence on programs, activities, costs and impact on health outcomes of using community health workers. World Health Organization; 2007. Acquired April 30, 2015 from: http://www.who.int/hrh/documents/community health workers.pdf.

[55] Viswanathan M, Kraschnewski J, Nishikawa B, Morgan LC, Thieda P, Honeycutt A, Lohr KN, Jonas D. Outcomes of Community Health Worker Interventions. Evidence Report/Technology Assessment No. 181 (Prepared by the RTI International–University of North Carolina Evidence-based Practice Center under Contract No. 290 2007 10056 I.) AHRQ Publication No. 09-E014. Rockville, MD: Agency for Healthcare Research and Quality. June 2009. Acquired April 30, 2015 from: http://www.ahrq.gov/research/findings/evidence-based-reports/comhworkevidence-report.pdf.

[56] Centers for Disease Control and Prevention. Policy Evidence Assessment Report: Community Health Worker Policy Components. Atlanta, GA: U.S. Department of Health and Human Services, Centers for Disease Control and Prevention; 2014. Acquired April 30, 2015 from: http://www.cdc.gov/dhdsp/pubs/docs/chw_evidence_assessment_report.pdf.

[57] Centers for Disease Control and Prevention. Addressing Chronic Disease through Community Health Workers: A Policy and Systems Level Approach. Second Edition. Atlanta, GA: U.S. Department of Health and Human Services, Centers for Disease Control and Prevention. 2015. Acquired April 30, 2015 from: http://www.cdc.gov/dhdsp/docs/chw_brief.pdf.

[58] Guide to Community Preventive Services. Cardiovascular disease prevention and control: interventions engaging community health workers. Acquired September 24, 2015 from: www.thecommunityguide. org/cvd/CHW.html.

[59] Dower C, Knox M, Lindler V, O'Neil E. Advancing Community Health Worker Practice and Utilization: The Focus on Financing. San Francisco, CA: National Fund for Medical Education. 2006. Acquired June 3, 2015 from: http://www.futurehealth.ucsf.edu/Content/29/2006-12_Advancing_Community_Health_Worker_Practice_and_Utilization_The_Focus_on_Financing.pdf.

[60] Medicaid and Children's Health Insurance Programs: Essential Health Benefits in Alternative Benefit Plans, Eligible Notices, Fair Hearings and Appeal Process, and Premiums and Cost Sharing, Exchange: Eligibility and Enrollment Federal Register. Acquired April 30, 2015 from: http://www.gpo.gov/fdsys/pkg/FR-2013-07-15/pdf/2013-16271.pdf.

[61] Update on Preventive Services Initiatives, CMCS Informational Bulletin; November 2013. Acquired April 30, 2015 from: http://medicaid.gov/Federal-Policy-Guidance/Downloads/CIB-11-27-2013-Prevention.pdf.

[62] Dower C, Knox M, Lindler V, O'Neil E. Advancing Community Health Worker Practice and Utilization: The Focus on Financing. San Francisco, CA: National Fund for Medical Education, 2006.

[63] Dower C, Knox M, Lindler V, O'Neil E. Advancing Community Health Worker Practice and Utilization: The Focus on Financing. San Francisco, CA: National Fund for Medical Education, 2006.
[64] Dower C, Knox M, Lindler V, O'Neil E. Advancing Community Health Worker Practice and Utilization: The Focus on Financing. San Francisco, CA: National Fund for Medical Education, 2006.
[65] Dower C, Knox M, Lindler V, O'Neil E. Advancing Community Health Worker Practice and Utilization: The Focus on Financing. San Francisco, CA: National Fund for Medical Education, 2006.
[66] Gates A, Rudowitz R, Guyer J. An Overview of Delivery System Reform Incentive Payment (DSRIP) Waivers. September 29, 2014. Acquired November 4, 2015 at: http://kff.org/medicaid/issue-brief/an-overview-of-delivery-system-reform-incentive-payment-waivers/.
[67] CMS – Medicaid Innovation Accelerator Program. Acquired November 4, 2015 at: http://www.medicaid.gov/State-ResourceCenter/Innovation-Accelerator-Program/innovation-accelerator-program.html.
[68] Our Mission. The CMS Innovation Center. Acquired July 30, 2015 from: http://innovation.cms.gov/About/Our-Mission/index.html.
[69] Personal Communication. CDR Thomas Pryor, BSN, U.S. Public Health Service. Preventive and Population Health Care Models Group, Center for Medicare and Medicaid Innovation and Ellen-Marie Whelan, NP, PhD., Acting Chief Population Health Officer, Center for Medicaid and CHIP Services (CMCS) and Senior Advisor, Center for Medicare and Medicaid Innovation (CMMI) and Centers for Medicare and Medicaid Services (CMS).
[70] Center for Medicare and Medicaid Innovation. State Innovation Models Initiative: Model Test Awards. Acquired June 3, 2015 from: http://innovation.cms.gov/initiatives/State-Innovations-Model-Testing/index.html.
[71] Center for Medicare and Medicaid Innovation. State Innovation Models Initiative: Model Test Awards Round Two. Acquired June 3, 2015 from: http://innovation.cms.gov/initiatives/state-innovations-model-testing-round-two/.
[72] Center for Medicare and Medicaid Innovation. Health Care Innovation Awards. Acquired June 3, 2015 from: http://innovation.cms.gov/initiatives/Health-Care-Innovation-Awards/Project-Profiles.html and http://inno vation.cms.gov/initiatives/Health-Care-Innovation-Awards/Round-2.html.
[73] Allen C, Brownstein JN, Jayapaul-Philip B, Matos S, Mirambeau A. Strengthening the Effectiveness of State-Level Community Health Worker Initiatives Through Ambulatory Care Partnerships. Journal of Ambulatory Care Management. July/September 2015. 38 (3): 254–262.
[74] Institute of Medicine. A Population-Based Policy and Systems Change Approach to Prevent and Control Hypertension. Washington, D.C.: National Academy of Sciences, 2010.
[75] Barbero C, Gilchrist S, Schooley MW, Chriqui JF, Luke DA, Eyler AA. Appraising the evidence for public health policy components using the quality and impact of component evidence assessment. Glob Heart 2015 Mar;10(1): 3-11.
[76] Medicaid and Children's Health Insurance Programs: Essential Health Benefits in Alternative Benefit Plans, Eligible Notices, Fair Hearings and Appeal Process, and

Premiums and Cost Sharing, Exchange: Eligibility and Enrollment Federal Register. Acquired April 30, 2015 from: http://www.gpo.gov/fdsys/pkg/FR-2013-07-15/pdf/2013-16271.pdf.
[77] Update on Preventive Services Initiatives, CMCS Informational Bulletin; November 2013. Acquired April 30, 2015 from: http://medicaid.gov/Federal-Policy-Guidance/Downloads/CIB-11-27-2013-Prevention.pdf.
[78] Personal Communication. Ellen-Marie Whelan, NP, PhD., Acting Chief Population Health Officer, Center for Medicaid and CHIP Services (CMCS) and Senior Advisor, Center for Medicare and Medicaid Innovation (CMMI) and Centers for Medicare and Medicaid Services (CMS).
[79] Dower C, Knox M, Lindler V, O'Neil E. Advancing Community Health Worker Practice and Utilization: The Focus on Financing. San Francisco, CA: National Fund for Medical Education, 2006.
[80] Alliance Creates Community Health Workers' Scope of Practice, Training Curriculum, Certificate Program, and Reimbursement Strategy, Expanding Their Integration Into the Health System to Reduce Health Disparities. Policy Innovation Profile. Innovation Exchange. Agency for Healthcare Research and Quality. Acquired June 3, 2015 from: https://innovations.ahrq.gov/profiles/alliance-creates-community-health-workersscope-practice-training-curriculum-certificate.
[81] Rosenthal EL, Brownstein JN, Rush CH, Hirsch GR, Willaert AM, Scott JR, Holderby LR, Fox DJ. Community health workers: part of the solution. Health Aff (Millwood). 2010 Jul; 29(7): 1338-1342.
[82] Dower C, Knox M, Lindler V, O'Neil E. Advancing Community Health Worker Practice and Utilization: The Focus on Financing. San Francisco, CA: National Fund for Medical Education, 2006.
[83] Dower C, Knox M, Lindler V, O'Neil E. Advancing Community Health Worker Practice and Utilization: The Focus on Financing. San Francisco, CA: National Fund for Medical Education, 2006.
[84] Medicaid.gov. Managed Care. Acquired June 3, 2015 from: http://medicaid.gov/medicaid-chip-program-information/by-topics/deliverysystems/managed-care/managed-care-site.html.
[85] Dower C, Knox M, Lindler V, O'Neil E. Advancing Community Health Worker Practice and Utilization: The Focus on Financing. San Francisco, CA: National Fund for Medical Education. 2006.
[86] Health Plus. Amerigroup. Acquired June 3, 2015 at: https://providers.amerigroup.com/Pages/NY.aspx.
[87] Dower C, Knox M, Lindler V, O'Neil E. Advancing Community Health Worker Practice and Utilization: The Focus on Financing. San Francisco, CA: National Fund for Medical Education, 2006.
[88] Gates A, Rudowitz R, Guyer J. An Overview of Delivery System Reform Incentive Payment (DSRIP) Waivers. September 29, 2014. Acquired November 4, 2015 at: http://kff.org/medicaid/issue-brief/an-overview-of-delivery-system-reform-incentive-payment-waivers/.
[89] Burton A, Chang DI, Gratale D. Medicaid Funding of Community-Based Prevention. Myths, State Successes Overcoming Barriers and the Promise of Integrated Payment Models. June 2013. Acquired June 3, 2015 from: http://www.nemours.org/content/

dam/nemours/wwwv2/filebox/about/Medicaid Funding of Community-Based Prevention Final.pdf.
[90] Burton A, Chang DI, Gratale D. Medicaid Funding of Community-Based Prevention. Myths, State Successes Overcoming Barriers and the Promise of Integrated Payment Models. June 2013. Acquired June 3, 2015 from: http://www.nemours.org/content/dam/nemours/wwwv2/filebox/about/Medicaid Funding of Community-Based Prevention Final.pdf.
[91] Burton A, Chang DI, Gratale D. Medicaid Funding of Community-Based Prevention. Myths, State Successes Overcoming Barriers and the Promise of Integrated Payment Models. June 2013. Acquired June 3, 2015 from: http://www.nemours.org/content/dam/nemours/wwwv2/filebox/about/Medicaid Funding of Community-Based Prevention Final.pdf.
[92] Dower C, Knox M, Lindler V, O'Neil E. Advancing Community Health Worker Practice and Utilization: The Focus on Financing. San Francisco, CA: National Fund for Medical Education, 2006.
[93] Family PACT. Acquired on June 3, 2015 from: http://www.familypact.org/.
[94] Dower C, Knox M, Lindler V, O'Neil E. Advancing Community Health Worker Practice and Utilization: The Focus on Financing. San Francisco, CA: National Fund for Medical Education, 2006.
[95] Dower C, Knox M, Lindler V, O'Neil E. Advancing Community Health Worker Practice and Utilization: The Focus on Financing. San Francisco, CA: National Fund for Medical Education, 2006.
[96] Blue Ridge Area Health Education Center (AHEC). http://www.vhwda.org/work force-development/regions/blue-ridge.

In: Community Health Workers
Editor: Cecilia Hodges
ISBN: 978-1-63485-060-5

Chapter 2

OUTCOMES OF COMMUNITY HEALTH WORKER INTERVENTIONS*

Meera Viswanathan, Jennifer Kraschnewski, Brett Nishikawa, Laura C. Morgan, Patricia Thieda, Amanda Honeycutt, Kathleen N. Lohr and Dan Jonas

STRUCTURED ABSTRACT

Objectives. To conduct a systematic review of the evidence on characteristics of community health workers (CHWs) and CHW interventions, outcomes of such interventions, costs and cost- effectiveness of CHW interventions, and characteristics of CHW training.

Data sources. We searched MEDLINE®, Cochrane Collaboration resources, and the Cumulative Index to Nursing and Allied Health Literature for studies published in English from 1980 through November 2008.

Review methods. We used standard Evidence-based Practice Center methods of dual review of abstracts, full-text articles, abstractions, quality ratings, and strength of evidence grades. We resolved disagreements by consensus.

Results. We included 53 studies on characteristics and outcomes of CHW interventions, 6 on cost-effectiveness, and 9 on training. CHWs interacted with participants in a broad array of locations, using a spectrum of materials at varying levels of intensity. We classified 8 studies as low intensity, 18 as moderate intensity, and 27 as high intensity, based on the type and duration of interaction.

Regarding outcomes, limited evidence (five studies) suggests that CHW interventions can improve participant knowledge when compared with alternative approaches such as no intervention, media, mail, or usual care plus pamphlets. We found mixed evidence for CHW effectiveness on participant behavior change (22 studies) and health outcomes (27 studies): some studies suggested that CHW interventions can result in greater improvements in participant behavior and health outcomes when compared

* This is an edited, reformatted and augmented version of a contracted report (AHRQ Publication No. 09-E014), issued by the U.S. Department of Health and Human Services, Agency for Healthcare Research and Quality, June 2009.

with various alternatives, but other studies suggested that CHW interventions provide no statistically different benefits than alternatives. Low or moderate strength of evidence suggests that CHWs can increase appropriate health care utilization for some interventions (30 studies). The literature showed mixed results of effectiveness when analyzed by clinical context: CHW interventions had the greatest effectiveness relative to alternatives for some disease prevention, asthma management, cervical cancer screening, and mammography screening outcomes. CHW interventions were not significantly different from alternatives for clinical breast examination, breast self-examination, colorectal cancer screening, chronic disease management, or most maternal and child health interventions.

Six studies with economic and cost information yielded insufficient data to evaluate the cost- effectiveness of CHW interventions relative to other community health interventions.

Limited evidence described characteristics of CHW training; no studies examined the impact of CHW training on health outcomes.

Conclusions. CHWs can serve as a means of improving outcomes for underserved populations for some health conditions. The effectiveness of CHWs in numerous areas requires further research that addresses the methodological limitations of prior studies and that contributes to translating research into practice.

EXECUTIVE SUMMARY

Introduction

The United States has experienced remarkable improvements in public health and medical progress throughout much of the twentieth century, including major advances in pharmaceutical and medical device innovation and gains in life expectancy. These improvements, however, have not been accessible to all parts of U.S. society. Substantial disparities in life expectancy, health, and health care persist. Although many actors—including health care systems, insurers, health care providers, and patients—contribute to these disparities, bias, discrimination, and stereotyping during the clinical encounter also explain health care disparities. Experts recommend reducing fragmentation in health care systems, improving awareness on the part of health care providers of these problems, strengthening culturally competent approaches to the delivery of health care, and increasing the diversity of the health care workforce, as strategies to reduce health care disparities. A core component in recommendations to address healthcare disparities is the involvement of the community: specifically, the involvement of community health workers (CHWs).

The RTI International–University of North Carolina at Chapel Hill Evidence-based Practice Center (RTI-UNC EPC) conducted a systematic review on outcomes of CHW interventions. The review addressed four key questions (KQs):

KQ 1. How do CHWs interact with participants? Specifically, what is the place of service, type of service, type of educational materials used, duration of interaction with participants, and length of followup?

KQ 2. What is the impact of CHWs on outcomes, particularly knowledge, behavior, satisfaction, health outcomes, and health care utilization?

KQ 3. What is known about the cost-effectiveness of CHWs for improving health outcomes?

KQ 4a. What are characteristics of training for CHWs in the outpatient setting?

KQ 4b. Are particular training characteristics associated with improved outcomes for patients?

Methods

We searched MEDLINE®, Cochrane Collaboration resources, and the Cumulative Index to Nursing and Allied Health Literature for studies published in English from 1980 through November 2008 in the United States. We refined KQs in collaboration with a panel of technical experts. We searched data sources using more than 10 terms for CHWs, including the Medical Subject Heading term "community health aides." We used standard Evidence-based Practice Center methods of dual review of abstracts, full-text articles, abstractions, quality ratings, and strength of evidence grades. We resolved disagreements by consensus. We identified 53 studies addressing KQ 1 and KQ 2, 6 studies addressing KQ 3, and 9 studies addressing KQ 4.

Results

KQ 1: Characteristics of Community Health Worker Interaction with Participants

KQ 1 asks for descriptions of the interaction between CHWs and participants; specifically, we examined place of service, type of service, type of educational materials used, duration of interaction with participants, and length of follow-up. CHWs interacted with participants in a broad array of locations, using a spectrum of materials at varying levels of intensity. Studies usually described the place of service and type of intervention in some detail. Across the studies, one-on-one interventions generally occurred in the home, over the telephone, or in a medical setting; by contrast, group interventions tended to take place in a community setting. Studies described types of educational materials poorly or not at all. Studies inconsistently reported duration of interaction with participants and length of followup (the number and length of sessions), and studies did not always clarify whether their reporting was based on protocol or on actual experience.

We synthesized the variety of ways in which CHWs can interact with participants into a single measure of intensity that serves as a proxy of resource allocation. We classified interactions that reported at least four of six elements suggesting a higher resource utilization (one-on-one, face-to-face, 1 hour per session or more, 3 or more months' duration, three or more interactions, and tailored materials) as high intensity; interventions with two or three elements as moderate intensity; and interventions with only one or none of the elements as low intensity. Of the total of 53 studies, we classified 27 as high intensity, 18 as moderate intensity, and 8 as low intensity. The intensity of CHW interventions varied by clinical context: maternal and child health and chronic disease management interventions were all moderate or high intensity, whereas prevention and screening studies were more likely to include low-intensity interventions.

KQ 2: Outcomes of Community Health Worker Interventions

KQ 2 asks about the impact of CHWs on outcomes, with specific attention to the following five domains: knowledge, behavior, satisfaction, health outcomes, and health care utilization. In addition, we summarize results by a key source of heterogeneity, the clinical context of the CHW intervention.

Summary by Outcomes

Knowledge. The five studies reporting information on knowledge together provided moderate strength of evidence that CHW interventions improve the knowledge of participants on disease prevention and cancer screening, compared with other alternatives, and provided low strength of evidence that CHW interventions improve knowledge of label reading among diabetics, compared with usual care, but these studies gave insufficient evidence for knowledge of other issues related to the management of diabetes. This literature did not compare CHWs with a comprehensive range of usual care providers; we cannot therefore conclude that CHWs outperform all alternatives in improving participant knowledge. For the small subset of comparators and outcomes included in this literature, the studies together suggest that CHW interventions can improve participant knowledge when compared with alternative approaches such as no intervention, media, mail, or usual care plus pamphlets.

Behavior. Twenty-two studies reported on the effect of CHW interventions on participant behavior. The evidence for workplace safety, diabetes mellitus, and the use of bedding encasements for asthma, from five studies, suggested that CHW interventions result in improvements in participant behavior when compared with alternatives such as a community intervention, a lower-intensity CHW intervention, and usual care combined with a pamphlet. The strength of evidence is moderate for the use of bedding encasements for asthma and low for workplace safety and diabetes mellitus. The evidence for disease prevention, improving the environment for child well-being, planned use of cancer screening tests, and breast self- examination, from 14 studies, is mixed, with some studies demonstrating a statistically significant benefit of the CHW arm, and others demonstrating a lack of significant difference. The strength of evidence for these outcomes is low. The evidence for health promotion among Latinas, injury prevention at home, and smoking cessation to reduce asthma, from five studies, failed to demonstrate that CHW interventions resulted in significantly different outcomes than alternatives; the strength of evidence for these outcomes is low.

Together these studies suggest that CHW interventions can, in some instances, result in greater positive changes in participant behavior when compared with a range of alternatives (including no intervention, community intervention, usual care plus a newsletter, media, print, a less intense or delayed CHW arm, or a combination of interventions). In other instances, CHW interventions provided no statistically different benefit when compared with a range of alternatives. When the alternative requires greater resource allocation, as with the use of health care professionals, the absence of statistically significant differences may favor the use of CHWs.

Satisfaction. A single study, focusing on mental health among the homeless, found no differences between study arms in participant satisfaction; the strength of evidence for this outcome is low.

Health outcomes. The literature examined CHW effectiveness on a range of outcomes: 27 of 53 studies reported health outcomes. Moderate strength of evidence exists that CHW interventions improve health outcomes for two clinical areas (improving back pain and improving psychosocial outcomes among caregivers of children with asthma) when compared with either a lower-intensity CHW intervention or a delayed-intervention control group (three studies). The evidence for other outcomes (pediatric immunizations, prenatal care and perinatal outcomes, child development, environment conducive to child well-being, mental health, diabetes, and asthma symptoms), from 22 studies, is mixed, with some studies suggesting that CHW interventions are more effective than alternatives (including no intervention, usual care, and nurses), and other studies showing no difference between CHW interventions and alternatives. For disease prevention (specifically, reduction in body mass index), hypertension, and mental health, the evidence from five studies suggests no difference between CHW interventions and alternative approaches, including the use of CHWs in a lesser capacity, nurses, and print materials; the strength of evidence for these outcomes is low.

Together these studies showed that CHW interventions had a greater effect on some health outcomes when compared with alternatives such as no intervention, usual care, and nurses, but these findings were not consistent across all studies; several studies found no statistically significant benefit of the CHW arm when compared with alternative approaches.

Health care utilization. More than one-half of the identified studies reported on health care utilization. Fifteen studies provided moderate strength of evidence that CHW interventions increase appropriate health care utilization for disease prevention, mammography, infectious diseases, and asthma when compared with a range of alternatives such as no intervention, mail, print, or a less intense CHW arm. Two studies offered low strength of evidence that CHW interventions provide statistically significant benefits in health care utilization for two outcomes: prenatal and perinatal care (when compared with nurses) and hypertension (when compared with usual care). For Pap smears, six studies provided mixed evidence, with some studies suggesting a statistically significant benefit for the CHW arm, and other studies suggesting no significant differences; the strength of evidence for this outcome is low. For health promotion among Latinas, child well-being, clinical breast examination, colorectal cancer screening, and mental health, evidence from nine studies suggested no difference between the CHW intervention and alternatives; the strength of evidence for these outcomes is low.

Together these studies provided low to moderate evidence that CHW interventions increase appropriate health care utilization (e.g., more use of cancer screening tests, less use of emergency services) when compared with a range of alternatives for disease prevention (specifically, medical follow-up for elevated blood pressure), mammography, infectious diseases, and asthma; for other reported outcomes, the evidence was mixed or does not show a statistically significant benefit of the CHW arm.

Summary Findings by Clinical Context

Health promotion and disease prevention. Eleven studies addressed health promotion and disease prevention, including pediatric immunizations, cardiovascular disease, diabetes prevention, HIV prevention, secondhand smoke exposure, colorectal cancer prevention, and general preventive care. Two studies on disease prevention found that CHW interventions versus print or no intervention were more effective in changing knowledge. Results for CHW interventions on behavior outcomes were mixed, with one-half of the studies favoring CHW intervention versus control groups, which consisted of no intervention, media, print, or a combination of interventions. None of the studies evaluated outcomes in the area of satisfaction. Results for CHW interventions on health outcomes, available from four studies, were also mixed.

The results suggest that CHW interventions may serve as an effective means of improving knowledge outcomes and possibly other outcomes related to preventing disease in underserved, minority populations.

Injury prevention. Three studies assessed injury prevention measures and associated behavioral outcomes: two focused on home injury prevention, and one considered workplace injury prevention. One study found improvements in behavior associated with CHW interventions when compared with a minimal community intervention, and one found mixed results with CHW interventions showing a statistically significant benefit in some measures but controls (with no intervention) showing a statistically significant benefit over CHW interventions for other measures. One study showed no significant difference in behavior between CHW interventions and health care professionals. The mixed results preclude any firm conclusions regarding the benefit of CHW interventions for injury prevention behaviors.

Maternal and child health. Fifteen studies meeting our inclusion criteria involved primarily maternal health, child health, or both and reported mainly on health outcomes. A statistically significant benefit of CHWs over standard care was shown most prominently in rapidity of metabolic control for mothers with phenylketonuria (PKU) and in the mental development of infants of mothers with PKU. CHW interventions were associated with a greater likelihood of initiating breastfeeding among African Americans, more frequent use of nonviolent discipline methods by parents, and higher parenting efficacy scores when compared with video- intervention or no-intervention controls. CHWs were also associated with significant attenuation in the decline of cognitive and motor development among infants with failure to thrive and with a lesser degree of increase in depressive symptoms among postpartum women when compared with no intervention. No significant advantage to CHW intervention was seen for improvements in incidence of low birth weight, presence of neonatal or infant health problems, language development, maternal stress or self-esteem, continuation of breastfeeding beyond 1 week, tobacco exposure for children of smokers, continued drug use among mothers with known prior drug use, growth of children with failure to thrive, or incidence of child maltreatment when compared with nurse interventions, multidisciplinary specialty clinical care, video or print intervention, routine health care, or no intervention.

Most studies involving CHWs for maternal and child health have been concerned with high- risk populations. For maternal and child health, CHWs appear to be most beneficial when addressing existing health conditions instead of potential conditions (i.e., primary prevention). Of the 15 studies that were evaluated, 8 studies reported statistically significant benefit to CHWs, compared with nurse interventions, multidisciplinary specialty clinical care, video or print intervention, routine health care, or no intervention. CHWs have not yet been shown to improve key health outcomes relating to maternal and child health such as prematurity, low birth weight, sustained breastfeeding, or child maltreatment relative to other alternatives such as video or print intervention, routine health care, or no intervention. The lack of such findings suggests that either further research is needed to demonstrate benefits or that there is a true lack of benefit for CHWs in this domain.

Cancer screening. Fifteen studies examining knowledge or health care utilization outcomes of CHW interventions for improving breast, cervical, or colorectal cancer screening met inclusion criteria for this systematic review. Together the 15 studies suggest limited evidence of improvement in knowledge in the CHW arm, compared with alternative approaches such as media or mail, and these studies also suggest conflicting findings on the effect of CHWs on planned or actual behavior changes—specifically, breast self-examination—when compared with no intervention, delayed intervention, mail, minimal CHW, or usual care. The volume of evidence on these outcomes is limited; the quality and design of the studies limit the interpretation of available evidence. Regarding health care utilization, our findings from limited evidence suggest that CHW interventions are not effective in comparison with other alternatives (such as no intervention, mail, tailored print and video, and minimal CHW) in raising the rates of clinical breast examination or colorectal cancer screening. More substantial evidence exists on Pap smears and mammography. The evidence suggests that the CHW arm is at least as effective as other alternatives (such as mail or lower-intensity CHW interventions) in improving Pap smear rates, but more effective than other alternatives (such as no intervention, media, print, community interventions, and usual care) only with low- and moderate-intensity interventions (rather than high-intensity interventions). Studies demonstrated significantly greater improvements in the CHW arm, compared with the alternative (no intervention, mail, print, or minimal CHW) in the main analysis or in subgroup analysis among low-income, minority, or other underserved subsamples.

CHW interventions were not demonstrated to be more effective than alternatives for increasing the utilization of breast self-examination, clinical breast examination, or colorectal cancer screening. CHWs can serve as a means of improving utilization of Pap smear tests and mammograms for underserved populations; the effectiveness of CHWs for other outcomes requires further research.

Chronic disease management. Thirteen studies addressed disease management, including diabetes mellitus, hypertension, asthma, back pain, mental health, and tuberculosis. Only one of the studies in the area of chronic disease management addressed knowledge outcomes. Two of four CHW interventions on diabetes and two asthma studies addressed behavior changes, comparing the CHW arm with usual care or a less intense CHW arm. These studies found that CHW interventions provided statistically significant benefit for diabetes and for use of bedding encasements in asthma, but not for smoking cessation. Only the mental health study addressed satisfaction outcomes, and this study did not demonstrate a difference between the CHW group and the control. Regarding health outcomes, two of four studies focusing on diabetes management found that a CHW intervention was more effective than usual care in decreasing hemoglobin A1c. None of the studies addressing hypertension management showed a significant difference in blood pressure control between groups. Two asthma studies demonstrated that CHW interventions were more effective than alternatives in reducing unscheduled health care services, improving psychological outcomes, and changing behavior, although symptom measures improved equally in each group. With the exception of asthma, the majority of CHW interventions for chronic disease management (specifically, diabetes, hypertension, and mental health) failed to show consistently greater improvement in health outcomes than usual care. By contrast, four of five studies on chronic disease management found that a CHW intervention was more effective than usual care or a less intense CHW arm in improving health care utilization.

KQ 3: Cost-Effectiveness of Community Health Worker Interventions

We identified six studies in the literature providing economic analyses of CHW interventions. All of the studies included in our review estimated intervention program costs, but not all reported the specific components of those costs or the year for which costs were estimated. None of the CHW intervention evaluations that included an economic analysis reported a standard measure of costs per quality-adjusted life year saved, as recommended in recent guides for performing economic evaluations. One study did report on the costs per life-year saved of the CHW intervention, but potential biases in measurement limit the interpretation of results. We found insufficient evidence to evaluate whether CHW interventions are a cost- effective alternative to clinical interventions to promote health and prevent disease.

KQ 4: Training of Community Health Workers

We found only nine studies meeting our inclusion criteria that described the training of CHWs. All included studies reported evidence of improvement in knowledge or skills, and many focused on aspects of training relevant to the specific health concern. Few reported on training for cultural competence, recruitment and retention process skills, intake and assessment, or protocol delivery. The failure to report on these elements presents a roadblock to identifying critical elements of a standardized curriculum applicable to all CHWs.

No studies reported on the effects of CHW training on health outcomes. The question of how to tailor CHW training to improve health outcomes is a significant gap for future studies to address.

Discussion

CHW interventions have the potential to address two fundamental imperatives for improving health care in the United States: the need to address substantial and persistent health care disparities, and the need to translate more research into practice. CHWs, by virtue of their role as a bridge to the health care system, can help to disseminate widely efficacious interventions to populations that rarely benefit from health care advances.

Evidence about the effectiveness of CHWs relative to other choices is, however, mixed. Some studies demonstrated statistically significant benefits of the CHW approach, compared with other choices; other studies showed mixed results or no statistically significant differences between study arms. For the latter studies, one explanation is a lack of true benefit of the CHW arm relative to other choices. In addition, the choice of controls (including health professionals and CHWs in a lesser capacity), inadequate study power, and the Hawthorne effect may explain the lack of significant differences between CHWs and alternatives. The variation in and inadequate reporting on components of CHW interventions limit assessments of whether high- intensity interventions deliver greater value than low- or moderate-intensity interventions.

We found limited evidence that suggests that CHW interventions can improve participant knowledge when compared with alternative approaches such as no intervention, media, mail, or usual care plus pamphlets. We found mixed evidence for CHW effectiveness on participant behavior change and health outcomes: some studies suggested that CHW interventions can result in greater improvements in participant behavior and health outcomes when compared with various alternatives, but other studies suggested that CHW interventions provide no statistically different benefits. Low or moderate strength of evidence suggests that CHWs can increase appropriate health care utilization for some interventions. The literature showed mixed results of effectiveness when analyzed by clinical context: CHW interventions had the greatest effectiveness relative to alternatives for some disease prevention, asthma management, cervical cancer screening, and mammography screening outcomes. CHW interventions were not significantly different from alternatives for clinical breast examination, breast self-examination, colorectal cancer screening, chronic disease management, or most maternal and child health interventions. We found insufficient evidence to evaluate the cost-effectiveness of CHW interventions relative to other public health interventions.

Our review suggests that CHWs may serve as a means of improving outcomes for underserved populations for some health conditions, as described above. Other health concerns require further research that addresses the methodological limitations of prior studies to fully evaluate the effectiveness of CHW interventions.

SECTION 1. INTRODUCTION

Background

Health Disparities in the United States

The United States experienced remarkable improvements in public health and medical progress throughout much of the twentieth century. These advances, which have continued into the twenty-first century, have been accompanied by significant increases in medical spending. In 2003, total health care spending reached approximately $1.7 trillion, accounting for nearly 16 percent of the gross domestic product [1]. An estimated 5.6 percent of total health care spending was on biomedical research, a proportion unmatched by any other country [2]. Some experts note associations between US expenditures on biomedical research and major advances in pharmaceutical and medical device innovation [2] and accompanying improvements in life expectancy [3].

These improvements have not been accessible to all parts of US society. Substantial disparities in life expectancy [4], health, and health care persist [5-9]. Repeated measures of disparities in quality of care and access to care since 2003 demonstrate, at best, only minor improvements [5-9] According to an Institute of Medicine (IOM) committee report, *Unequal Treatment*, these seemingly intractable differences cannot be explained by clinically appropriate care, differing needs of patients, or patient preferences [10]. Moreover, access-related factors such as insurance status and income also cannot alone explain differences in quality of care or outcomes [10].

Although many actors, including health care systems, insurers, health care providers, and patients, contribute to these disparities, bias, discrimination, and stereotyping during the clinical encounter also explain health care disparities [10]. Recommendations of the IOM report, echoed by other publications [11, 12], focus on reducing fragmentation in health care systems, improving awareness on the part of health care providers of these problems, strengthening culturally competent approaches to the delivery of health care, and increasing the diversity of the health care workforce [10].

Role of the Community Health Worker in Addressing Health Disparities

A core component in recommendations to address health disparities is the involvement of the community, specifically the involvement of community health workers (CHWs) [10]. Models of care using CHWs vary from making them an integral part of the care delivery team to involving them as community navigators, education providers, or outreach agents [13].

A key variable along this spectrum is the extent to which CHWs operate within their own social networks. For example, CHW interventions using natural helpers rely on the specialized knowledge and expertise of CHWs working within their own social networks, whereas an outreach worker model may operate across social networks [14]. The nomenclature for CHWs reflects this variation; it includes terms such as natural helpers, lay health advisors, patient navigators, and community health aides, among others. The disease conditions that CHWs help to address also reflect a wide spectrum, from AIDS prevention to smoking cessation, hypertension management to pediatric immunization, and asthma management to maternal and child care.

Common attributes across CHWs, regardless of nomenclature, health condition, or intervention include: (1) their role as health workers who share a relationship with their community (e.g., shared language, ethnicity, geography, race, or disease condition) and (2) the absence of professional training. The relationship that CHWs share with the community in which they work has long identified them as a natural bridge to the health care system.

Explanations for the anticipated outcomes of CHW interventions typically cite theories of individual behavior change [15-23]. Theories of individual behavior change draw upon many ideas. Among them are the stages of change or the transtheoretical model (a framework for understanding motivational readiness to address problem behaviors [24]), social learning or social cognitive theory (an explanation of individual learning as operating through the observation of others within the context of behavioral, environmental, and personal factors [25]), and the health belief model (an explanation of individual health behaviors through attitudes and beliefs toward perceived susceptibility, severity, benefits, and barriers [26]).

Less frequently, authors acknowledge that these interventions also operate within the context of community change [27-29]. According to Minkler and Wallerstein, collaborative models of community change range from community organizing (externally driven and motivated by community needs) to community building (internally generated and drawing upon community strengths) with variants in between [30]. Several ideas help explain the drivers and mechanisms of community change: theories of social justice and human rights (the idea of health as a human right that CHWs can help to achieve in the interest of social justice [28, 31]), collaborative empowerment (grantmakers, support organizations, local leaders, and individuals working together in a reciprocal manner [32]), and critical consciousness (the process of critical awareness by which community members become aware of their own agency and create spaces to work with others to bring about changes in individual and community health [33, 34]).

CHW engagement is expected to diffuse community change to individuals; in addition, CHWs are postulated to reduce disparities through improving access to care, providing culturally competent health education, counseling, and sometimes rendering direct health services. Additionally, as trusted members of the community, CHWs may help to minimize barriers to care resulting from health beliefs and health values [10].

History of Community Health Workers

The history of CHWs supports the role that they continue today in providing services to marginalized populations. Perez and Martinez [28] note that the earliest records of CHWs date back to a shortage of doctors in early 17th century Russia, when lay people, called "feldshers," received training to provide basic medical care to military personnel [35]. Later a similar model arose in China, where farmers with minimal medical training served as "barefoot doctors" to provide basic primary care, including vaccinations and treatment of minor illnesses, to rural underserved regions [28]. Today, thousands of health programs employ CHWs worldwide for similar reasons [36].

Internationally, a global shortage of medical workers has increased the call for these types of personnel. Significant health care workforce shortages are present in 57 countries, including countries in sub-Saharan Africa, Bangladesh, India, and Indonesia [37] Figures for the number of physicians per 100,000 people range from a low of 2 in Malawi to a high of 591 in Cuba; the number in the United States is 256 [37]. These figures represent overall physician proportions; the proportion of primary care physicians is far lower worldwide.

The AIDS epidemic in developing countries that already face a critical shortage of professional health care workers has strengthened the need to make greater use of CHWs. Task shifting allows CHWs to take on jobs that were previously performed by nurses; this phenomenon holds promise for rapidly filling the health care workforce deficit. One advantage of employing CHWs is the relatively short amount of training time they need, ranging from hours to weeks. This quick turnaround in training allows CHWs to be ready to provide services years before new nurses or doctors can complete their own training. Ultimately, the hope is that task shifting will improve access to primary care and, thus, serve to strengthen health care systems around the world [37].

In the United States, despite the relatively high ratios of physicians to patients in this country, a significant percentage of the population remains underserved, particularly for primary care. An estimated one in five Americans are medically disenfranchised due to the shortage of primary care physicians, meaning they have inadequate or even no access to these physicians [38]. The need to reduce health disparities among the underserved has led to an interest in CHW interventions within the United States. The 2007 Community Health Worker National Workforce Study suggests that the development of the CHW workforce in the United States occurred over four important time periods: early documentation (1966-1972), utilization of CHWs in special projects (1973-1989), state and federal initiatives (1990-1998), and public policy options (1999-2007) [13]. Few references to CHW interventions appear in the literature before the mid-1960s.

During the period of early documentation (1966-1972), CHWs were used to address problems of the poor rather than in specific health improvement models. The New York City Health Department first documented CHW use in a 1960s-era tuberculosis program that involved "neighborhood health aides." [39]. One early effectiveness study on CHWs (published in 1970) consisted of a CHW intervention with nurses and physicians to improve compliance in treating pediatric infections [40].

Public and private funding of projects involving CHWs continued to grow from 1973 to 1989, in turn prompting more publications [13]. Further attention was brought to CHWs as a result of a World Health Organization (WHO) declaration in 1978, proposing the development of national CHW programs as important for promoting primary health care [41]. Another significant step for dissemination of CHW programs occurred when the "Resource Mothers" curriculum, prepared for the Virginia Task Force on Infant Mortality during the 1980s, became one of the early CHW curricula distributed nationally [42].

From 1990 to 1998, several state and federal bills proposed CHW interventions; none, however, was enacted. Despite this lack of legislative support, training centers dedicated to CHWs opened in Boston [43] and San Francisco [44]. Support remained high for the promise of CHW interventions with the expectation that the widespread incorporation of CHWs into the health delivery system would offer opportunities to improve the delivery of preventive and primary health care in the United States [45].

The state of Texas passed the first legislation addressing the CHW workforce in 1999, starting the public policy options period (1999-2006) [13, 46]. During this time, several associations called for expansion of CHW roles and projects, including the National Rural Health Association, the American Association of Diabetes Educators, and the American Public Health Association. As noted earlier, the 2003 IOM report also made recommendations regarding the role of CHWs in addressing health care disparities [10]. Finally, during this same period the first national legislation on CHWs was passed: The Patient Navigator Outreach and Chronic Disease Prevention Act of 2005. Additionally, the state of Minnesota passed legislation allowing for Medicaid coverage of CHW services in December of 2007 [47].

In 2000, an estimated 86,000 CHWs were supporting American communities [13]. The number of CHWs has continued to grow since then to an estimated 121,000 CHWs in 2005, representing a 41 percent increase from 2000 [13].

Key Questions and Analytic Framework

Key Questions

Numerous recent reviews have examined the effectiveness of CHWs, but their scope has often been limited to specific disease conditions [48, 49] subpopulations [50, 51], or study designs [52, 53] The Agency for Healthcare Research and Quality (AHRQ) commissioned the RTI International– University of North Carolina Evidence-based Practice Center (RTI-UNC EPC) to conduct a systematic review on outcomes of CHW interventions. The nominator for this work was the Minnesota Department of Human Services (MDHS).

The EPC received and revised key questions (KQs) after discussions with internal technical staff, AHRQ staff, MDHS staff, and our Technical Expert Panel (TEP, see below). The final KQs are as follows:

KQ 1. How do community health workers interact with participants? Specifically, what is the place of service, type of service, type of educational materials used, duration of interaction with participants, and length of followup?

KQ 2. What is the impact of community health workers on outcomes, particularly knowledge, behavior, satisfaction, health outcomes, and health care utilization?

KQ 3. What is known about the cost-effectiveness of community health workers for improving health outcomes?

KQ 4a. What are characteristics of training for community health workers in the outpatient setting?

KQ 4b. Are particular training characteristics associated with improved outcomes for patients?

Analytic Framework for Outcomes of Community Health Worker Interventions

Based on our discussion with TEP members, we used the following operational definition of CHWs: A CHW:

- Performs health-related tasks to create a bridge between community members, especially hard-to-reach populations, and the health care system (i.e., performs tasks extending beyond peer counseling or peer support alone).
- Has health training associated with the intervention; training is shorter than that of a professional worker (i.e., training does not form part of a tertiary education certificate).
- Is recognized (or can be identified) as a member of the community in which he or she works, defined by but not limited to, geographic location, race or ethnicity, and exposure or disease status.

As reflected in Figure 1, KQ 1 and KQ 4a are descriptive questions. The information obtained through KQ 1 will inform KQ 2. KQ 3 evaluates cost information for the subset of evidence identified in KQ 1 as effective. The heterogeneity of health conditions, CHW intervention types, and comparators will be explicitly addressed in all KQs.

Production of This Evidence Report

Organization

Section 2 describes our methods, including our search strategies and inclusion/exclusion criteria; we also document our approach to grading the quality of articles and rating the strength of evidence. In Section 3, we report the results of literature searches and synthesis of retained articles for KQs 1, 2, 3, and 4. Section 4 presents our conclusions and offers our recommendations for future research.

References and included studies follow Section 4. Appendixes include a detailed description of our search strings (Appendix A), data collection forms (Appendix B), detailed evidence tables (Appendix C), excluded studies (Appendix D), and acknowledgments (Appendix E).

Technical Expert Panel (TEP)

In designing the study questions and methodology at the outset of this report, we consulted several technical and content experts, seeking broad expertise and perspectives. We identified seven technical experts to provide assistance throughout the project (Appendix E); two were employed by the Minnesota Department of Human Services (the nominator for this topic). The TEP contributed to AHRQ's broader goals of (1) creating and maintaining science partnerships as well as public-private partnerships and (2) meeting the needs of an array of potential customers and users of its products. Thus, the TEP was both an additional resource and a sounding board during the project.

Divergent and conflicting opinions are common; we perceive them as healthy scientific discourse that contributes to a thoughtful, relevant systematic review. Nonetheless, in the end, study questions, design, and/or methodologic approaches do not necessarily represent the views of individual technical and content experts.

To ensure robust, scientifically relevant work, we called on the TEP to provide reactions to work in progress and advice on substantive issues or possibly overlooked areas of research. Specifically, TEP members participated in conference calls and discussions through e-mail to:

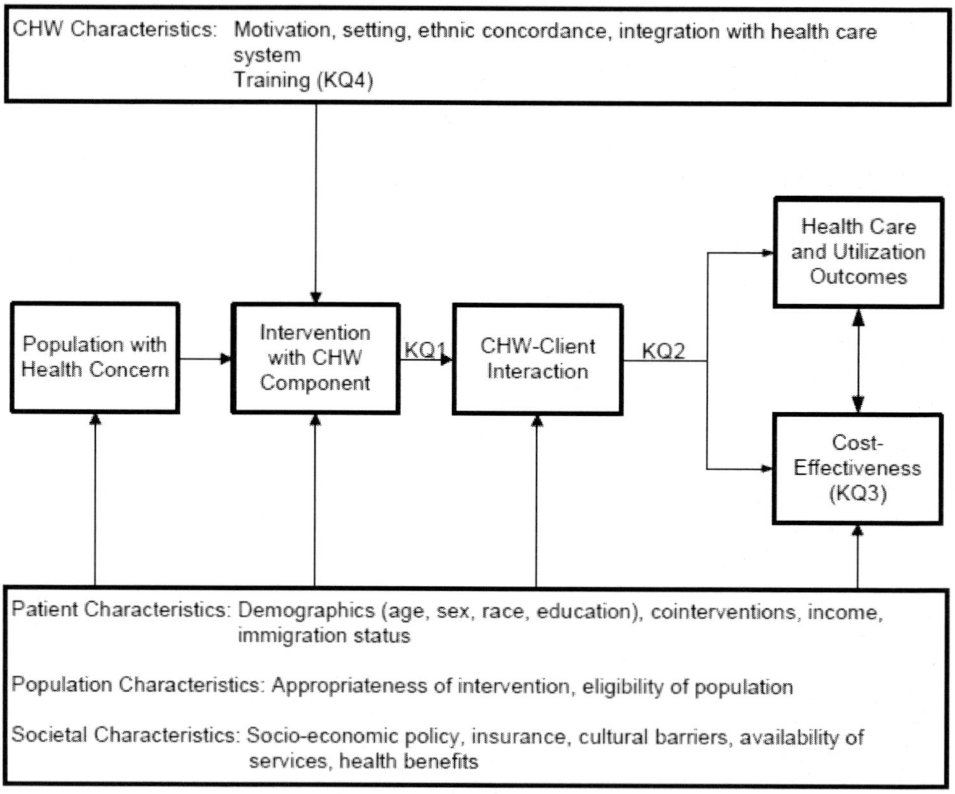

Figure 1. Outcomes of community health worker interventions: conceptual framework.

- refine the analytic framework and KQs at the beginning of the project;
- discuss the preliminary assessment of the literature, including inclusion/exclusion criteria; and
- provide input on the information and categories included in evidence tables.

Because of their extensive knowledge of the literature, including numerous articles authored by TEP members themselves, and their active involvement in the field, we also asked TEP members to participate in the external peer review of the draft report.

Uses of This Report

We anticipate that this report will be useful to primary care and public health practitioners; community health workers; national, state, and local health policy makers; Medicaid and other public and private insurers; and community-based researchers. As noted above, we will explicitly consider CHW effectiveness by clinical concern; specialists in these areas may also find this report to be of use in designing and allocating resources for future CHW interventions.

SECTION 2. METHODS

In this section, we document the procedures that the RTI International–University of North Carolina Evidence-based Practice Center (RTI–UNC EPC) used to develop this comprehensive evidence report on community health workers (CHWs). The team was led by a senior health services researcher (Meera Viswanathan, Ph.D., Study Director), and included a physician trained in internal medicine and pediatrics (Dan Jonas, M.D., M.P.H.), a general internist (Jennifer Kraschnewski, M.D.), a preventive medicine physician (Brett Nishikawa, M.D.), an economist (Amanda Honeycutt, Ph.D.), and two EPC staff members, Laura Morgan, M.A., and Patricia Thieda, M.A.

We describe our inclusion and exclusion criteria, search and retrieval process, and methods of abstracting relevant information from the eligible articles to generate evidence tables. We also discuss our criteria for grading the quality of individual articles and for rating the strength of the evidence as a whole.

Literature Review Methods

Inclusion and Exclusion Criteria

Our inclusion and exclusion criteria are documented in Table 1. As noted in Section 1, this systematic review focuses on characteristics, outcomes, cost-effectiveness, and training of CHWs. We restricted our searches to the United States so that we could have data relevant to domestic health care concerns. We also restricted our searches to studies published in 1980 or thereafter to ensure that results had relevance to current practice.

We excluded studies that (1) were published in languages other than English (given the available time and resources); (2) did not report information pertinent to the key clinical questions; (3) had fewer than 40 subjects for randomized controlled trials (RCTs) or nonrandomized cohorts with comparisons; and (4) were not original studies.

A key criterion for inclusion was the requirement that the effect of the CHW had to be abstractable. As a result of this criterion, our review is limited to studies for which the effect of the CHW intervention can be isolated; we excluded 38 studies in which the outcome of the intervention could not be attributed to the CHW. These studies often compared usual care to a combination of interventions that may have included CHWs as one of several components and did not distinguish between the effect of the CHW and other components. Another key criterion was the requirement that the intervention included CHWs. As a result, we excluded studies that relied on peer counselors (13 studies).

For key questions (KQs) 1, 2, and 3, we required that the CHW intervention be compared with an alternative; we excluded 70 studies without comparison arms. For KQ 4, we required that the description of training for CHWs be supported by pre- and post-training evaluation data; we excluded 34 studies without such data.

Table 1. Inclusion/exclusion criteria

Category	Criteria
Populations	All study populations with a CHW intervention
Interventions	Intervention must be delivered by CHWs, not peer counselors or healthcare professionals. A CHW: • Performs health-related tasks to create a bridge between community members, especially hard-to-reach populations, and the health care system (i.e., performs tasks extending beyond peer counseling or peer support alone). • Has health training associated with the intervention; training is shorter than that of a professional worker (i.e., training does not form part of a tertiary education certificate). • Is recognized (or can be identified) as a member of the community in which he or she works, defined by but not limited to, geographic location, race or ethnicity, and exposure or disease status.
Comparisons	KQs 1, 2, 3: CHW intervention must have a comparison arm; all comparisons admissible as long as the effect of the CHW intervention can be abstracted KQ 4: No comparisons required
Outcomes	KQ 1: Interaction with clients KQ 2: Knowledge, satisfaction, behavior, health outcomes, and health care utilization KQ 3: Cost data KQ 4: Training characteristics
Time period	1980 to November 14, 2008
Study settings and geography	United States
Publication languages	English only
Admissible evidence (study design and other criteria)	**Admissible designs** controlled trials (n $\geq$40), nonrandomized controlled trials (n $\geq$40), systematic reviews, meta-analyses, prospective trials with historical controls (n $\geq$40) **Other criteria** • Original research studies must provide sufficient detail regarding methods and results to enable use and adjustment of the data and results • Relevant outcomes must be able to be abstracted from data presented in the papers • Effect of CHW intervention must be abstractable • KQ 4: CHW interventions must provide pre-training and post-training evaluation of CHW knowledge or skills

Table 2. MEDLINE search strategy and unduplicated results for April 2008

Search number	Search Term	Yield
#2	Search "Community Health Aides" [MeSH] OR "health advisor" OR "health worker" OR "health advocate" OR "health paraprofessional" OR "community health representative" OR "outreach worker" OR dumas OR promotor as OR embajadores OR consejeras	6,051
#3	Search "Community Health Aides "[MeSH] OR "health advisor" OR "health worker" OR "health advocate" OR "health paraprofessional" OR "community health representative" OR "outreach worker" OR dumas OR promotoras OR embajadores OR consejeras Limits: Humans, English	3,031
#6	Search (("Outcome Assessment (Health Care)" [MeSH] OR "Pregnancy Outcome" [MeSH])) OR ("Treatment Outcome"[MeSH] OR "Outcome and Process Assessment (Health Care)" [MeSH] OR "Fatal Outcome" [MeSH]) Limits: Humans, English	369,350
#7	Search #3 AND #6 Limits: Humans, English	175
#17	Search ("Patient Education as Topic" [MeSH] OR "Patient Education Handout "[Publication Type]) OR "Professional-Patient Relations" [MeSH]) OR "Office Visits" [MeSH] Limits: Humans, English	109,582
#18	Search #3 AND #17 Limits: Humans, English	90
#26	Search ("Costs and Cost Analysis" [MeSH] OR "Economics" [MeSH] OR "economics "[Subheading] OR "Cost-Benefit Analysis" [MeSH] OR "Cost Allocation"[MeSH] OR "Cost of Illness" [MeSH] OR "Cost Control" [MeSH] OR "Cost Sharing" [MeSH] OR "Cost Savings" [MeSH] OR "Health Care Costs" [MeSH] OR "Direct Service Costs" [MeSH] OR "Hospital Costs" [MeSH] OR "Employer Health Costs" [MeSH] OR "Drug Costs" [MeSH]) Limits: Humans, English	257,114
#27	Search #3 AND #26 Limits: Humans, English	254
#28	Search United States Limits: Humans, English	606,881
#29	Search #27 AND #28 Limits: Humans, English	71
#33	Search (("Education"[MeSH] OR "education "[Subheading])) OR "Education, Professional"[MeSH] OR training Limits: Humans, English	370,579
#34	Search #3 AND #33 Limits: Humans, English	1,013
#35	Search #34 AND #28 Limits: Humans, English	241
#41	Search ("Randomized Controlled Trials as Topic" [MeSH] OR "Randomized Controlled Trial "[Publication Type]) OR "Single-Blind Method" [MeSH]) OR "Double-Blind Method" [MeSH]) OR "Random Allocation" [MeSH] Limits: Humans, English	303,728
#42	Search #3 AND #41 Limits: Humans, English	165
#44	Search control OR controlled Limits: Humans, English	1,368,901
#45	Search #3 AND #44 Limits: Humans, English	908
#46	Search #45 AND #28 Limits: Humans, English	154
	Total unduplicated PubMed records	640

Literature Search and Retrieval Process

Databases. We searched three electronic databases—MEDLINE®, Cochrane Collaboration resources, and Cumulative Index to Nursing and Allied Health Literature (CINAHL). We also hand-searched the reference lists of relevant articles to make sure that we did not miss any relevant studies. We consulted with our Technical Expert Panel (TEP) about any studies or trials that were currently under way or that had not yet been published.

Table 3. Overall unduplicated results and sources of all searches

Original search of MEDLINE, Cochrane, Cochrane Clinical Trials Registry, CINAHL (April 2008)	809
Update search of MEDLINE, Cochrane, Cochrane Clinical Trials Registry, CINAHL (November 2008)	59
TEP recommended references	10
Handsearches of reference lists	173
Supplemental search (Patient Navigator) of MEDLINE, Cochrane, Cochrane Clinical Trials Registry, CINAHL	25
TOTAL	1,076

Search terms. Based on the inclusion/exclusion criteria above, we generated a list of Medical Subject Heading (MeSH) search terms (Table 2 and Appendix A). Our TEP also reviewed these terms to ensure that we were not missing any critical areas, and this list represents our collective decisions as to the MeSH terms used for all MEDLINE searches.

Our initial searches in MEDLINE produced 640 unduplicated records. Searches in other databases (CINAHL, Cochrane, and Cochrane Clinical Trials Registry) yielded 169 new records (unduplicated across all databases) for a total of 809 records. We conducted update searches in all databases in November, 2008 and supplemented electronic searches with manual searches of reference lists. In addition, we received recommendations for studies of interest from the TEP and conducted a supplemental search on patient navigators after peer review. In all, we identified 1,076 unduplicated references from all searches (Table 3).

Figure 2 presents the yield and results from our searches, which we conducted from April through November 2008. Beginning with a yield of 1,076 articles, we retained 89 articles that we determined were relevant to address our KQs and met our inclusion/exclusion criteria (Figure 2). We reviewed titles and abstracts of the articles against the basic inclusion criteria above; we retained relevant articles and used them as appropriate in the discussion in Section 4.

Article selection process. Once we had identified articles through the electronic database searches, review articles, and reference lists, we examined abstracts of articles to determine whether studies met our criteria. Each abstract was independently, dually reviewed for inclusion or exclusion, using an Abstract Review Form (Appendix B). If one reviewer concluded that the article should be included in the review, we retained it.

Of this entire group of 1,076 citations, 590 required full review. For the full article review, one team member read each article and decided whether it met our inclusion criteria, using a Full-Text Inclusion/Exclusion Form (Appendix B). Reasons for article exclusion are listed in Appendix D.

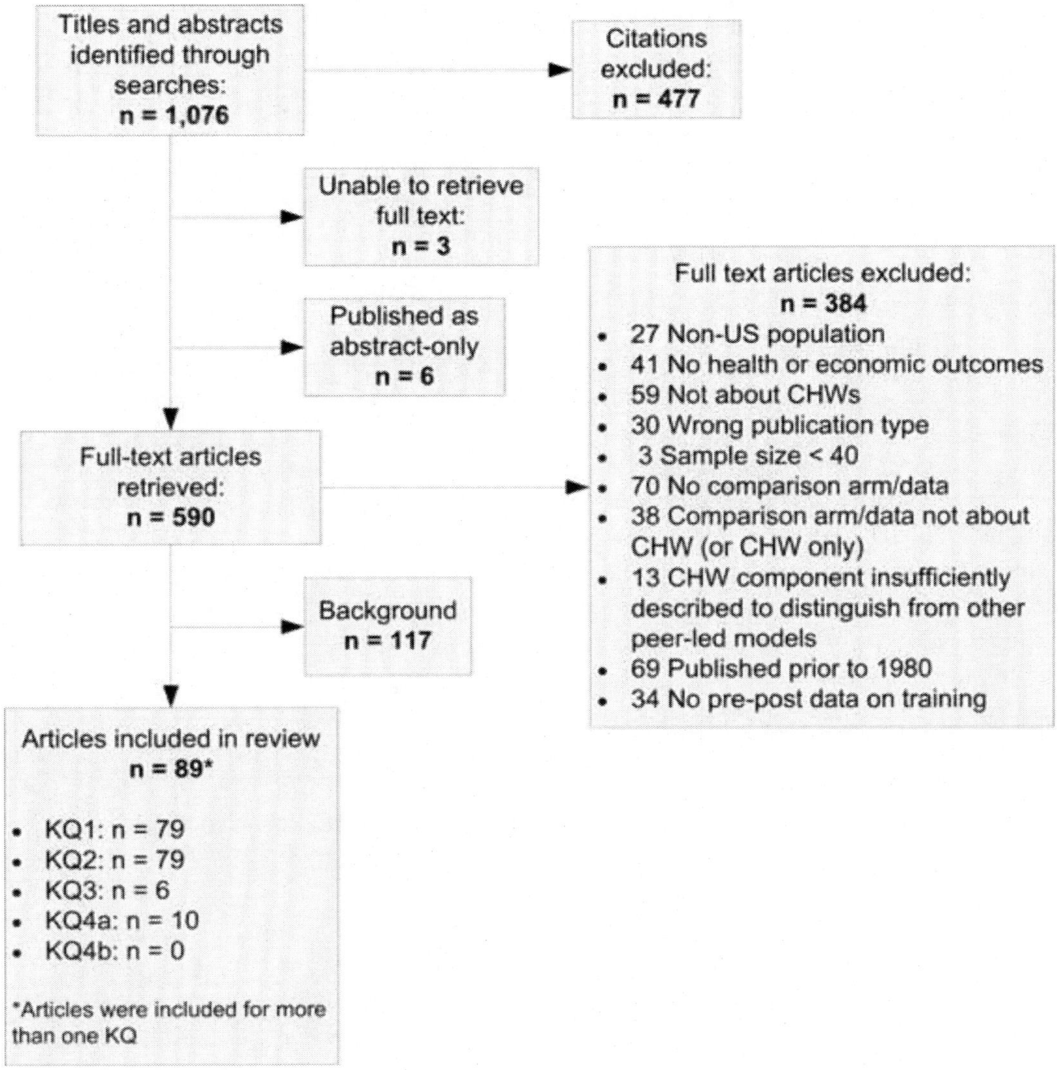

Figure 2. Results of literature search.

Literature Synthesis

Development of Evidence Tables and Data Abstraction Process

The team jointly developed the evidence tables. We designed the tables to provide sufficient information to enable readers to understand the studies and to determine their quality; we gave particular emphasis to essential information related to our KQs. We based the format of our evidence tables on successful designs that we have used for prior systematic reviews.

Table 4. Strength of evidence grades and definitions

Grade	Definition
High	High confidence that the evidence reflects the true effect. Further research is very unlikely to change our confidence in the estimate of effect.
Moderate	Moderate confidence that the evidence reflects the true effect. Further research may change our confidence in the estimate of effect and may change the estimate.
Low	Low confidence that the evidence reflects the true effect. Further research is likely to change our confidence in the estimate of effect and is likely to change the estimate.
Insufficient	Evidence either is unavailable or does not permit estimation of an effect.

We trained abstractors by having them abstract several articles into evidence tables and then reconvening as a group to discuss the utility of the table design. The abstractors repeated this process through several iterations until they decided that the tables included the appropriate categories for gathering the information contained in the articles.

Four members of the team (Jennifer Kraschnewksi, Brett Nishikawa, Laura Morgan, and Patricia Thieda) shared the task of initially entering information into the evidence tables. Authors of individual sections reviewed the articles and edited all initial table entries for accuracy, completeness, and consistency. Abstractors reconciled all disagreements concerning the information reported in the evidence tables. The full research team met regularly during the article abstraction period and discussed global issues related to the data abstraction process.

The final evidence tables are presented in their entirety in Appendix C. Studies are presented in the evidence tables alphabetically by the last name of the first author. A list of abbreviations and acronyms used in the tables appears at the beginning of that appendix.

Quality Rating of Individual Studies

Quality rating forms for RCTs have been validated and in use for several years; a similarly well-validated form for observational studies does not exist. RTI has been developing a form to rate observational studies [54]. This form, which can be used to rate the quality of a variety of observational studies, was based on a review of more than 90 AHRQ systematic reviews that included observational studies; we supplemented this review with other key articles identifying domains and scales [55, 56]. We structured the resultant form largely on the basis of the domains and subdomains suggested by Deeks and colleagues; [55] we then adapted it for use in this systematic review (Appendix B).

The form currently includes review of nine key domains for observational studies: background, sample selection, specification of exposure, specification of outcome, soundness of information, followup, analysis comparability, analysis of outcome, and interpretation. An additional domain for RCTs is the quality of randomization. We used these dimensions of quality to assess the overall quality of the study. We did not attempt to construct a quantitative scale for quality. Previous scales have been critiqued for their lack of inter-rater reliability. An additional concern is scales do not account for a single flaw that may substantially bias results, despite meeting standards for all other aspects of study quality. Each study was dually evaluated for quality; abstractors reconciled all disagreements.

Strength of Available Evidence

We evaluated the strength of evidence based on the AHRQ Comparative Effectiveness Methods Guide [57]. The strength of evidence for each outcome incorporates risk of bias, consistency, directness, precision, and the presence of other modifying factors. As described in Owens et al., the evaluation of risk of bias includes assessment of study design and aggregate quality of studies [57]. We judged good quality studies with strong designs to result in evidence with low risk of bias. We graded evidence as consistent when effect sizes across studies were in the same direction and had a narrow range. When the evidence linked the interventions directly to health outcomes, we graded the evidence as being direct. We graded evidence as being precise when results had low degree of uncertainty. When considering the effect of confounders, we evaluated whether the degree of intensity of interventions in both arms could have explained the effects (or absence of effects); additionally we considered whether other sources of effect modification or confounding had been accounted for. We dually evaluated the overall strength of evidence for each outcome based on a qualitative assessment of strength of evidence for each domain and reconciled all disagreements. The levels of strength of evidence are shown in Table 4.

Applicability of the Evidence

We evaluated the applicability of the evidence based on a qualitative assessment of the population, intensity, or quality of treatment, choice of the comparator, outcomes, and timing of followup. We based our parameters for evaluation on guidance provided by AHRQ's Comparative Effectiveness Methods Guide [58]. Specifically, we consider whether enrolled populations differ from target populations and how this might affect risk of benefits or harms, whether studied interventions compare to those in routine use and how this might affect risk of benefits or harms, whether comparators reflect best alternative treatment and how this may influence treatment effect size, whether measured outcomes are known to reflect the most important clinical benefits and harms, and whether followup is sufficient to detect clinically important benefits.

External Peer Review

AHRQ's Scientific Resource Center requested review of this report from a wide array of outside experts. We received three external reviews and revised the report as appropriate.

Section 3. Results

This section presents the results of our evidence review for the following four key questions (KQs): KQ 1, interaction of CHWs with participants; KQ 2, outcomes of community health worker (CHW) interventions; KQ 3, cost-effectiveness of CHW interventions; and KQ 4, training of CHWs and the relationship between CHW training and patient health outcomes. We note that KQ 3, on cost-effectiveness of CHW outcomes, is derivative of KQ 2 and is limited to studies demonstrating effectiveness. As noted in Section 2, a total of 53 studies qualified for inclusion for KQ 1 and KQ 2, 6 for KQ 3, and 9 for KQ 4.

Appendix C-1provides the detailed evidence tables for KQs 1, 2, and 3. Appendixes C-2 and C-3 present individual quality ratings for randomized clinical trials (RCTs) and observational studies, respectively. Appendix C-3 provides detailed abstractions for KQ 4. All evidence tables are presented in alphabetical order by last name of the first author.

As noted in earlier sections, an overall assessment of the effectiveness of CHW outcomes requires evaluation of sources of heterogeneity, including clinical context, intensity of interaction between CHWs and participants, and type of comparator. CHW interventions operate in a variety of clinical contexts; summarizing the effects of these interventions on varied outcomes requires an explicit consideration of the clinical context. For this reason, we have organized the results for KQs 1, 2, and 3 by the clinical context of the interventions identified. These are, specifically, health promotion and disease prevention, injury prevention, maternal and child health, cancer screening, and chronic disease management.

An additional source of heterogeneity is the degree of intensity of the intervention, which can vary by clinical context. We synthesize the evidence from KQ 1 to develop a measure of the intensity (low, moderate, or high) of the interaction between CHWs and participants, and we then include the measure in describing results for KQ 2 and KQ 3. We also record other sources of heterogeneity such as the type of comparator. Section 4 discusses the effectiveness of CHW interventions and the potential impact of sources of heterogeneity on effectiveness more fully.

This literature is characterized by several articles together constituting a single study. We refer to studies in the text and cite all relevant articles for each study; article and study counts, therefore, frequently do not match. Our summary tables below feature groups of studies addressing each outcome. Unless otherwise stated, these tables are organized alphabetically by the last name of the first author. The summary tables for KQ 2 and KQ 3 provide information to identify the study (author, and date of publication), study design, population and setting, sample size, study quality, intervention and comparators, and results.

KQ 1: Interaction of Community Health Workers and Participants

KQ 1 focuses on how CHWs interact with participants, specifically the place of service, type of service, type of educational materials used, duration of interaction with participants, and length of contact. We categorize place of service as over the telephone or based in the clinic, the community, home, or workplace. Interventions often employed multiple settings to interact with participants. The type of services ranged from one-on-one interactions to group interactions. All CHW interventions included some element of education; we sought to understand the degree to which these materials were standardized or tailored for each participant. We identified three elements of duration of interaction: the number of sessions, time per session, and the length of time from the first interaction to the last interaction (length of contact). We report summary findings below, for each descriptor, of the interaction between CHWs and participants across all studies and clinical contexts. These characteristics vary greatly across CHW interventions, but a common element is the overall intensity of the intervention. Interventions of lower intensity will require fewer resources than interventions of moderate or high intensity. As a proxy measure of resource allocation, we employ characteristics of the CHW-participant intervention to develop a measure of intensity of interaction. As noted earlier, a key organizing principle for understanding the effectiveness of

CHW interventions is clinical context; we conclude this section by describing characteristics of CHW-participant interactions and their intensity by clinical context. Summary tables describing the characteristics of CHWs are provided by clinical context; within each table, studies are presented in order of intensity and then in alphabetical order, by the last name of the first author.

Overview of Interaction between Community Health Workers and Participants

Place of service. CHWs interacted with participants over the telephone or provided services in one or more of four locations: home, community, clinic, or workplace. CHWs provided home, telephone, and clinic interventions on a one-on-one basis; community interventions were more likely to be oriented toward groups than to individuals. Thirty-two studies had at least one home visit but may have involved telephone and community components as well [15, 17, 18, 23, 59-102]. Interventions in five studies occurred primarily by telephone [19-22, 69, 70, 103-106]. In nine studies, interventions included at least one meeting in a community setting and were primarily group- oriented [27, 59, 60, 107-115]. Interventions taking place in the community generally occurred in churches [59, 60, 107, 108] or in other neighborhood or community locations [27, 102, 109-114, 116-122]. Eight studies involved community interventions but did not specify the location; [27, 109-115, 118-120] of these, only two were one-on-one interventions [118-121]. One intervention occurred in a neighborhood beauty salon [116], and four occurred on the street or in shelters [117-122] Five studies took place within clinics or health care settings [23, 77, 99, 123-125]. One intervention occurred in the workplace [126]. We could not determine the place of service for one intervention [16, 127].

Type of service. The type of services varied greatly across included studies. CHWs provided a wide range of services including one-on-one counseling (face-to-face and by telephone), education, support, information on health and community resources, transportation, appointment reminders, and other forms of assistance. The type of service ranged from brief one-time interactions to intensive one-on-one interactions over a span of years. The minimal service provided was a brief, one-time interaction such as distributing condoms and providing prevention literature [117] or a single telephone call to promote cancer screening [103]. At the other end of the spectrum, many interventions had multiple face-to-face counseling sessions, often in the home, to address specific needs.

Type of educational materials used. The least described characteristic of the interaction between CHWs and clients is the type of educational material used. As many as twenty-seven studies did not report any details on the type of educational materials utilized [16, 19-23, 67-74, 78, 79, 83, 85-92, 96, 97, 99, 101, 104-108, 117, 120-122, 124, 125, 127]. Several studies did not describe educational materials per se but did report that they distributed "materials" as part of the intervention (e.g., safety glasses, materials to reduce exposure to asthma triggers, smoke detectors). The remainder provided minimal descriptions that ranged from the use of a postcard [66] to complex systems, including audio and written formats to appeal to the broadest range of subjects [63]

Duration of interaction (time per session and number of sessions). The duration of interaction varied broadly overall. Interactions lasted from quite brief (5 minutes to an hour) one- time meetings to extensive multiple interactions totaling several hours in all.

Length of contact. The length of contact—that is, the length of time that CHWs were directly involved with participants (which may have differed from the length of the study, or the length of time between measurement of pre- and postintervention health outcomes)—was inadequately reported in many cases. Length of contact ranged from 1 day [15, 103, 108, 116, 117] to 2.5 years [98].

Intensity of Interaction

Based on the type of interaction, the duration of interaction (time per session, number of sessions, and length of interaction), and the tailoring of CHW interactions, we classified the intensity of an intervention into three categories: low, moderate, or high. Interactions that had at least four of six elements suggesting a higher intensity (one-on-one, face-to-face, an hour per session or more, 3 or more months' duration, three or more interactions, and tailored materials) were classified as high intensity. Interventions with two or three elements were classified as moderate intensity. Interventions with only one or none of the elements were classified as low intensity.

In making these classifications, we relied, whenever possible, on the protocol intentions rather than what actually occurred. When no information was available for the protocol, we relied on reported interactions in the field. When interactions in the field were also not reported, we assumed lower intensity for that aspect for the intervention. For instance, when studies did not report the time spent in each session, we assumed that the time per session did not exceed an hour on average. Similarly, if studies did not report specifically that the materials were tailored for each participant, we assumed that the interventions used generic materials for all participants.

Low-intensity interventions were generally one-time interactions, usually in a group setting. Moderate-intensity interventions occurred in a variety of settings but typically involved only one or two interactions with CHWs over shorter periods of time. High-intensity interventions included multiple interactions, face-to-face, for 3 months or more. Each category varies internally: for instance, within the high-intensity interventions, the number of interactions could vary from 3 to more than 20 in a year, depending on the nature of the intervention. Of the total of 53 studies, we classified 8 studies as low intensity [19-22, 59, 60, 103, 104, 107, 108, 113, 117, 126], 18 as moderate intensity [106, 125, 15, 23, 63, 66, 69, 70, 99, 101, 102, 105, 109-112, 114, 116, 118, 119, 122-124] and 27 as high intensity [16-18, 27, 61, 62, 64, 65, 67, 68, 71-98, 100, 120, 121, 127, 128].

Community Health Worker-Participant Interaction by Clinical Context

Community health worker-participant interactions for health promotion and disease prevention intervention. We included 11 studies on health promotion and disease prevention (Table 5). Six studies occurred in the home and by telephone; [64-71] one additional study was by telephone and mail [105]. Three studies were conducted in community settings—one in anonclinical site [118, 119], one in churches [107], and one on community streets [117]. For one study, the place of service was not reported [16, 127]. The majority of studies did not report the educational materials used; one of these studies provided condoms as part of the intervention [117] Only four studies provided some description of the educational materials used during the intervention [64-66, 117-119]

Five studies were of high intensity [16, 64, 65, 67, 68, 71, 127], four of moderate intensity [66, 69, 70, 105, 118, 119], and two of low intensity [107, 117].

Community health worker-participant interactions for injury prevention interventions. We included three studies in injury prevention (Table 6) [101, 102, 126]. Two took place primarily in the home [101, 102] and one on farms [126]. Two studies involved the distribution of materials to improve safety; [102, 126] one study did not report the educational materials used [101]. Two studies were of moderate intensity; [101, 102] one was of low intensity [126].

Community health worker-participant interactions for maternal and child health interventions. Overall we included 15 studies in maternal and child health (Table 7). All of the studies occurred primarily in the home, but 1 had opportunities for interactions in health care clinics [77]. Only 4 studies provided some description of educational materials used during the intervention; [75-77, 80-82, 84] the remaining 11 did not report any details [67, 68, 71-74, 78, 79, 83, 85-87, 128]. All the maternal and child health studies were of high intensity.

Table 5. CHW-participant interactions for health promotion and disease prevention

Author, Date of Publication	Place of Service	Type of Service	Educational and Other Materials Provided	Number of Sessions, Time per Session, and Length of Contact with Participants	Intensity—Low, Moderate, High
Auslander et al., 2002[16] Williams et al., 2001[127]	NR	Counseling adults for diabetes prevention: group and individual sessions	NR	6 group sessions and 6 individual sessions weekly, 45-90 minutes per session, over 3 months	High
Barnes et al., 1999 [68]	Home and telephone	Information and assistance, referral, transportation to clinic if needed for childhood immunizations	NR	Unspecified number of calls and visits, over 6 months (time per session NR)	High
Barnes-Boyd et al., 2001 [71] Nacion et al., 2000 [72]	Home	Family-focused care plan; support, model problem-solving skills, promote self-development of mother, provide instruction in infant care; transportation; find community resources for childhood immunizations	NR	12 monthly visits, over 1 year (time per visit NR)	High
Conway et al., 2004 [67]	Home and telephone	Problem-solving techniques to reduce environmental tobacco smoke exposure to children	NR	6 home and telephone visits over 4 months (time per session NR)	High

Table 5. (Continued)

Author, Date of Publication	Place of Service	Type of Service	Educational and Other Materials Provided	Number of Sessions, Time per Session, and Length of Contact with Participants	Intensity—Low, Moderate, High
Elder et al., 2005 [64] Elder et al., 2006 [65]	Home and/or telephone	Home visits or phone calls for Latinas to make healthful dietary behavior changes	Tailored newsletters with homework assignments	12 home visits or telephone calls over a 12-week period, 12 weekly tailored newsletters (time per session NR)	High
Becker et al., 2005 [118] Cene et al., 2008 [119]	Community--nonclinical site	Counseling for adults with risk factors for cardiovascular disease	Written, culturally sensitive	Multiple (number unspecified) 30-minute sessions over 1-year period	Moderate
Hunter et al., 2004 [66]	Home	Facilitated appointment scheduling for annual preventive exams for Latinas	Postcard	1 initial home visit and 1 final followup visit 8 weeks after postcard mailing to begin intervention (time per session NR)	Moderate
Krieger et al., 1999 [105]	Telephone and mail	Referral to medical care; appointment scheduling assistance; appointment reminder letter; followup to determine whether the appointment was kept; a new appointment for each missed appointment (up to 3); and assistance in reducing barriers to care through referral to community transportation, child care, or other services	NR	Various, brief interactions over 3 months (time per session NR)	Moderate
Rask et al., 2001 [69] LeBaron et al., 2004 [70]	Home and telephone	Appointment reminder, assistance in overcoming barriers to appointment for pediatric immunizations if needed	NR	At least 1 telephone call, followed by repeat calls and home visit if no telephone contact, over 15 months or less (time per interaction NR)	Moderate
Campbell et al., 2004 [107]	Community – churches	Provide information through existing networks; organize and conduct at least three church-wide activities focused on spreading information for colorectal cancer prevention	NR	3 church- based activities during 12 months (time per session NR)	Low
Wendell et al., 2003 [117]	Community—streets	Interview on sexual disease risk factors and prevention in at-risk adults; survey interaction	Condoms	Brief one-time interaction handing out condoms and prevention literature (time of interaction NR)	Low

NR, not reported.

Community health worker-participant interaction for cancer screening interventions. Overall 15 studies concerned cancer screening: 7 took place primarily in the home (visits or telephone) [15, 17-22, 61-63, 103, 104, 106] and 8 in community locations [59, 60, 107-113, 116, 125] (Table 8).

Table 6. CHW-participant interactions for injury prevention

Author, Date of Publication	Place of Service	Type of Service	Educational and Other Materials Provided	Number of Sessions, Time per Session, and Length of Contact with Participants	Intensity—Low, Moderate, High
Gielen et al., 2002[101]	Home	Assessed home for injury hazards such as falls, burns, and poisonings; made recommendations about appropriate safety products and practices; referred families to the Child Safety Center	NR	1 home-safety visit sometime between the patient's 6- and 9-month well-infant visits (time of session NR)	Moderate
Schwarz et al., 1993[102]	Home and community	Recruitment of volunteer representative from each block to identify neighborhood resources, facilitate contacts with residents, and reinforce safety messages through monthly block meetings. Home safety inspections in the presence of residents consisting of provision of safety materials; instruction on correcting safety hazards, simple household repairs, use of ipecac and bathwater thermometer, safety behaviors; identification of community resources	Safety materials: smoke detectors, batteries, bathwater thermometer, nightlight, ipecac, sticker for telephone with emergency numbers, and a poster with information on preventing burns, poisonings, falls, and injury from domestic violence	1 home visit and monthly block meetings over 18-month period (time per session NR)	Moderate
Forst et al., 2004[126]	Workplace (farms)	Distribution of eyewear, training on use and on eye health and safety	Reference manual on agricultural eye illness and injury; enlarged photos and fotonovelas; tool kit to demonstrate eye injuries and hazards; protective eyewear	At least 1 individual and at least 1 group session during farming season (time per session NR)	Low

NR, not reported.

Nine studies described some of the materials used during the intervention; [15, 17, 18, 59-63, 103, 109-113] six did not report the educational materials used [19-22, 104, 106-108, 116, 125]. We found two studies of high intensity [17, 18, 61, 62], seven of moderate intensity [15, 63, 106, 109-112, 116, 125] and six studies of low intensity [19-22, 59, 60, 103, 104, 107, 108, 113].

Community health worker–participant interactions for chronic disease management interventions. Overall, 13 studies focused on chronic disease management (Table 9). Seven took place primarily in the home [23, 88-100], 2 in health care settings [123, 124] and 4 in community locations [27, 114, 120-122]. Eight described some of the materials used during the intervention; [27, 93-98, 100, 114, 123] five did not report the educational materials used [23, 88-92, 99, 120-122, 124]. Two studies provided materials to households to reduce exposure to asthma triggers (bedding, vacuum cleaners, etc.) [96, 97, 100]. Eight were of high intensity [27, 88-98, 100, 120, 121] and five studies were of moderate intensity [23, 99, 114, 122-124].

Table 7. CHW-participant interactions for maternal and child well-being

Author, Date of Publication	Place of Service	Type of Service	Educational and Other Materials Provided	Number of Sessions, Time per Session, and Length of Contact with Participants	Intensity—Low, Moderate, High
Barnes-Boyd et al., 2001 [71]	Home	Family-focused care plan; support, model problem-solving skills, promote self-development of mother, provide instruction in infant care; transportation; find community resources	NR	Monthly visits over 12 months (time per session NR)	High
Barnes et al., 1999 [68]	Home and telephone	Information and assistance, referral, transportation to clinic if needed for childhood immunizations	NR	Unspecified number of calls and visits over 6 months (time per session NR)	High
Barth et al., 1988 [73]	Home	Task-directed approach to reduce risk of parenting problems including transportation, support and assistance with participant needs, advocating on participant's behalf, modeling positive parenting and homecare skills	NR	≈2 visits per month, ≈4 hours per session, over 6 months	High
Barth et al.,1991 [74]	Home	Task-directed approach to reduce the risk of parenting problems	NR	On average 11 visits (range 5-20) over 6 months (time per session not reported but ≈4 hours implied)	High

Author, Date of Publication	Place of Service	Type of Service	Educational and Other Materials Provided	Number of Sessions, Time per Session, and Length of Contact with Participants	Intensity—Low, Moderate, High
Black et al., 1995[75] Hutcheson et al., 1997 [76]	Home	Develop individualized family service plan with specific goals; support mother's needs; promote maternal-child relationship	Handouts, developmental assessment toys	Weekly visits (≈1 hour per visit) for 1 year	High
Caulfield et al., 1998 [77]	Community (WIC clinics), home or telephone	One-on-one counseling on participants' attitudes toward infant feeding, correcting misconceptions, group support sessions on infant feeding	Breastfeeding motivational video, posters and pamphlets	3 or more meetings during pregnancy (from 24 weeks of gestation) and then weekly up to 16 weeks postpartum if they continued breast feeding (time per meeting NR)	High
Conway et al., 2004 [67]	Home and telephone	Problem-solving techniques to reduce environmental tobacco smoke exposure to children	NR	6 home and telephone visits over 4 months (time per session NR)	High
Duggan et al., 1999 [78] Duggan et al., 2000 [128]	Home	Building relationships with families; active assistance to address existing crises; model problem-solving skills and effective parent-child interaction; link families with needed resources; provide parenting education; ensuring presence of medical home for children	NR	≈22 visits (1 hour each) over 2 years	High
Graham et al., 1992[79]	Home	Psychosocial support; educate family about pregnancy; advocate; link to community services for stress reduction; information on health risks during pregnancy and on nutrition	NR	4 visits (1 hour each) at 2-4 week intervals for 2-5 months (until birth of child)	High
Nacion et al., 2000 [72]	Home	Intensive home visits for assessment, problem-solving, emotional support, and information	NR	NR	High
Olds et al., 2002 [80] Korfmacher et al., 1999 [81] Olds et al., 2004 [82]	Home	Intensive home visitation: promoting healthy behaviors, competent child care, pregnancy planning, education, employment, linking to social and health services; promoting healthy	Visit-specific protocol, adapted to individual needs of mother	Every other week (except for weekly visits during the first 4 weeks after enrollment and the first 6 weeks after delivery) through the child's 21st month, followed by	High

Table 7. (Continued)

Author, Date of Publication	Place of Service	Type of Service	Educational and Other Materials Provided	Number of Sessions, Time per Session, and Length of Contact with Participants	Intensity—Low, Moderate, High
		family/friend relationships		monthly visits during the final 3 months, ≈75 minutes per sessionl	
St. James et al., 1999 [83]	NR (most likely home, based on activities like cooking)	Counseling, meal planning, pregnancy education, shopping, discuss medical recommendations	NR	≈20 sessions of 2 hours each (weekly in beginning then less frequently) throughout pregnancy	High
Schuler et al., 2000 [84]	Home	Teaching and counseling on infant development, health education, mother-infant interaction	Activity sheets	Weekly visits (mean duration 30.1 minutes per visit) for 6 months	High
Silver et al., 1997 [85]	Home	Counseling; share information on child health and behavior; link families with existing community resources	NR	6 meetings (1 hour each) with at least biweekly telephone calls and 3 group social activities over 12 months	High
Tessaro et al., 1997 [86] Navaie-Waliser et al., 2000 [87]	Home	Counseling, assistance in applying for government benefits, housing, employment, education, general advocacy for families	NR	One visit per month (more if needed) for approximately 14 months (time per visit NR)	High

≈, approximately; NR, not reported; WIC, Special Supplemental Nutrition Program for Women, Infants, and Children.

KQ 2: Outcomes of Community Health Worker Interventions

KQ 2 asks about the impact of CHWs on outcomes, particularly knowledge, behavior, satisfaction, health outcomes, and health care utilization. As noted earlier, the effect of CHW interventions will vary by clinical context (e.g., diagnosis or health concern), so as with KQ 1, we present results by clinical context for each of the outcomes described above. The areas of clinical concern are health promotion and disease prevention, injury prevention, maternal and child health, cancer screening, and chronic disease management.

We also assessed each study for quality; in general, we present results for higher quality studies first, followed by findings for moderate and then lower quality studies. We also give the level of intensity of the interaction between CHWs and participants and the type of comparator for each study, using the three intensity categories introduced in KQ 1. As noted there, the intensity of the interaction between CHWs and participants varied by clinical context. For example, maternal and child health interventions were solely high intensity whereas cancer screening studies ranged across high, medium, and low intensity. Because of this variation for cancer screening, we discuss those studies categorized first by intensity, then by quality. For all other clinical contexts, we did not find meaningful patterns by intensity of intervention, either because of lack of variation in intensity, or because the number of studies was insufficient to draw conclusions.

Table 8. CHW-participant interactions for cancer screening

Author, Date of Publication	Place of Service	Type of Service	Educational and Other Materials Provided	Number of Sessions, Time per Session, and Length of Contact with Participants	Intensity—Low, Moderate, High
Paskett et al., 2006 [17] Katz et al., 2007 [18]	Home and telephone	Education and barrier-specific counseling to promote screening; scheduling assistance	Individualized health education program	2 visits at 45-60 minutes and 30-45 minutes, 2 intervening telephone calls, and a final visit (time of final visit NR) over 9 to 12 months	High
Sung et al., 1997 [61] Sung et al., 1992 [62]	Home	Education on breast and cervical cancer, breast self-exam, educational materials on screening, facilitation to address logistical barriers to screening	Video of Pap and breast exam; printed materials	3 visits (months 1, 2, 4) over 4-month period, visits 1 and 2 for 1.5 hours each, time for visit 3 NR	High
Dignan et al., 200515	Home	Barrier-specific counseling to promote screening	Tailored brochure	One-time session of 20-90 minutes	Moderate
Hiatt et al., 1995 [125]	Community (various locations)	One-on-one support; education: contact with clients was ongoing and personal	NR	Unspecified # of interactions (time per interaction NR) over 2 years	Moderate
Jandorf et al., 2005 [106]	Telephone	One-on-one support and education on screening techniques and barriers to screening; assistance scheduling procedures	NR	At least 3 telephone calls (time per call NR) over 6 months	Moderate
Mock et al., 2007 [109]	Community	2 small group gatherings and individual direct contacts to help access medical services and schedule appointments	Language-specific flip charts and booklets	2 sessions of 90 or 120 minutes each over 3 to 4 months	Moderate
Navarro et al., 1995, 1998, 2000 [110-112]	Community	12 weekly small group educational sessions	Pamphlets, worksheets, posters developed for project and pamphlets from other organizations	12 sessions of 90 minutes each over 3 months	Moderate
Taylor, et al., 2002 [63]	Home and telephone	Tailored responses to individual barriers to cervical cancer	Video, motivational pamphlet,	One-time visit with followup telephone call (time per interaction NR)	Moderate

Table 8. (Continued)

Author, Date of Publication	Place of Service	Type of Service	Educational and Other Materials Provided	Number of Sessions, Time per Session, and Length of Contact with Participants	Intensity—Low, Moderate, High
		screening, clinic referral and scheduling assistance, translation services, transportation assistance	educational brochure, fact sheet, tailored counseling		
Wilson et al., 2008 [116]	Community—beauty salon	Education, counseling, and information on location of screening services during salon appointment	Written materials (not described)	1 visit (time of session NR)	Moderate
Andersen et al., 2000 [103]	Telephone	Barrier-specific telephone counseling to promote screening	Standardized script	1 interaction (time of interaction NR)	Low
Campbell et al., 2004 [107]	Community—churches	Provide information through existing networks; organize and conduct at least 3 church-wide activities focused on spreading information	NR	3 church-based activities during 12 months (time per session NR)	Low
Derose et al., 2000 [19] Duan et al., 2000 [20] Derose et al., 2000 [21] Fox et al., 1998 [104] Stockdale et al., 2000 [22]	Telephone	Barrier-specific telephone counseling to promote screening, discussion of resources for free- and reduced-cost mammograms, translation services, transportation, and childcare assistance	NR	2 telephone calls (1 per year over 2 years), time per session 7-11 minutes on average	Low
Earp et al., 2002 [113]	Community	Presentations to community groups and events; one-on-one conversations; use of informational/ motivational materials	Brochures, posters, church fans, holiday cards	2 community activities per month; one-on-one conversations once a week over a 24-month period, time per session NR	Low
Erwin et al., 1997 [108]	Church	Motivational speeches based on cancer survivor experience of CHWs, breast self-exam lessons using a breast model, discussion of resources for free- and reduced-cost mammograms	NR	1 presentation, time NR	Low
Sauaia et al., 2007 [59] Welsh et al., 2005 [60]	Community (church) and home	Personal education sessions to deliver health promotion messages	Newsletter	At least bimonthly meetings (time per meeting NR) over 5 years	Low

NR, not reported.

Table 9. CHW-participant interactions for chronic disease management

Author, Date of Publication	Place of Service	Type of Service	Educational and Other Materials Provided	Number of Sessions, Time per Session, and Length of Contact with Participants	Intensity—Low, Moderate, High
Batts et al., 2001 [88] Gary et al., 2003 [89] Gary et al., 2005 [90] Gary et al., 2000 [91] Vetter et al., 2004 [92]	Home and telephone	Offer to schedule appointments and visits, provide education, mobilize social support for adults with diabetes mellitus	NR	3 visits (45-60 minutes each) per year over 2 years (and additional contacts as needed)	High
Beckham et al., 2008 [93]	Home or clinic (site chosen by participant; majority preferred home)	Diabetes self-management education; referrals to registered dieticians, healing center	Visual aids (majority of participants illiterate)	Up to 15 home visits over 1 year, lasting 1-1.5 hours per visit	High
Frate et al., 1985 [94] Frate et al., 1983 [95]	Home or community	Monitor blood pressure; provide health education and support; self-management of hypertension for adults	Pamphlets, scale, low-salt cookbook, AHA and NHLBI pamphlets	Monthly visits over 18 months (time per session NR)	High
Krieger et al., 2005 [96] Krieger et al., 2002 [97]	Home	Environmental assessment; individualized action plan; education and social support; deliver materials to reduce trigger exposure for asthma	Materials to reduce asthma-trigger exposure	4 to 9 visits over 12 months (time per session NR)	High
Levine et al., 2003 [98]	Home	Education, counseling, referrals, providing information on access to health care, answered questions for adults with hypertension	Wallet-sized blood pressure tracking card, educational pamphlet	6 visits over 2.5 years (time per visit NR)	High
Lujan et al., 2007 [27]	Community (classroom), telephone, and mail	Deliver participative classes for adults with diabetes mellitus, answered questions, reinforce education, promote behavior change, send biweekly postcards	Audiovisual teaching aids (flip charts, food models, food labels) and handouts	8 weekly 2-hour classes + biweekly telephone calls for 8 weeks followed by biweekly postcards for 16 weeks 24 weeks' total duration of interaction with participants	High
Morse et al., 1997 [120] Wolfe et al., 1997 [121]	Community—unspecified locations (homeless population)	Assistance with activities of daily living and leisure activities for	NR	Face-to-face meetings (time per meeting and number NR) over 18 months	High

Table 9. (Continued)

Author, Date of Publication	Place of Service	Type of Service	Educational and Other Materials Provided	Number of Sessions, Time per Session, and Length of Contact with Participants	Intensity—Low, Moderate, High
		homeless people with psychiatric diseases			
Parker et al., 2008 [100]	Home	Environmental assessment; asthma action plan based on allergy tests; education and social support; mattress covers, pillows, vacuum, cleaning supplies; counseling on environmental tobacco smoke; integrated pest management services	Asthma booklet; materials to reduce asthma trigger exposure	At least 9 visits over 12 months (time per session NR)	High
Bone et al., 1989 [123]	Emergency room and telephone	Measured pulse and blood pressure (in emergency room session); provided educational counseling; identified barriers related to referrals, appointment keeping, and adherence to the treatment plan for adults with hypertension	Wallet-sized BP record card	1 face-to-face session (≈20 minutes) and at least 1 pre-followup appointment reminder telephone call (5-10 minutes) (time period over which this occurred NR)	Moderate
Corkery et al., 1997 [124]	Hospital clinic	Liaison between patients and health care providers for adults with diabetes mellitus; attended clinic sessions with patient; provided translation, appointment reminders; rescheduled missed appointments; reinforced self-care instructions	NR	Varied (mean = 3.4 months, range: 0.9-5.4), time per session equal to clinic visit duration	Moderate
Morisky et al., 2002 [23] Ward et al., 2000 [99]	Home and/or clinic	Counseling regarding lifestyle, medication-taking, and appointment-keeping; tailored to patient need for adults with hypertension	NR	Number of visits, time per session, time period over which interactions occurred NR	Moderate
Pilote et al., 1996 [122]	Community—shelters (homeless population)	Transported participants to clinic appointment for homeless people	None	Met participants and went to clinic within a 3 week period (time per session NR)	Moderate

Author, Date of Publication	Place of Service	Type of Service	Educational and Other Materials Provided	Number of Sessions, Time per Session, and Length of Contact with Participants	Intensity—Low, Moderate, High
		with tuberculosis; assisted with paperwork and doctor's recommendations			
Von Korff et al., 1998 [114]	Community—unspecified locations	Led classes on self-managing back pain, discussed strategies and barriers to achieve goals for managing pain	Book, pamphlets, videotapes, flipcharts	4, 2-hour classes held once a week for 1 month	Moderate

NR, not reported.

Variation in aims and clinical contexts of the studies, populations and settings, measures of health outcomes, and health care utilization information precluded quantitative synthesis of the results of studies. As with other questions, the number of articles exceeds the number of distinct studies. In all cases, tables list studies by quality (good, fair, then poor) and then alphabetically by last name of the first author of the article(s).

Outcomes for Health Promotion and Disease Prevention

Health promotion and disease prevention: pediatric immunizations. *Study characteristics.* Two RCTs, one good [69, 70] and one fair quality [68], and one poor-quality prospective cohort study (REACH-Futures [71, 72]) examined outcomes of CHW interventions to improve pediatric immunization rates in inner cities (Table 10). The RCTs used moderate-intensity interventions and the cohort study used a high-intensity intervention.

Both RCTs used CHWs to provide reminder telephone calls for upcoming clinic appointments. The good-quality RCT, targeting children < 12 months of age in a county public health clinic in metropolitan Atlanta, had CHWs make home visits only if a child remained behind on his or her immunization schedule [69, 70]. Additionally, this study compared four groups of children receiving: (1) automated telephone call reminders, (2) CHW outreach, (3) a combination of a CHW and automated telephone call reminders, and (4) a control group defined by normal clinic procedure [69, 70]. Outcomes were assessed after 22 months [69, 70].

The fair-quality trial, targeting low-income children in Manhattan, also used CHWs to provide basic immunization education and referral, in addition to assisting in obtaining immunization services through a combination of telephone and home visits [68]. It compared outcomes after 6 months for children receiving the CHW intervention with those for a control group comprising parents who were informed of their child's immunization status at enrollment and instructed to reschedule the missed appointment [68].

REACH-Futures, a prospective cohort study, compared a group receiving a high-intensity intervention of CHW and nurse visits with historic controls of nurse-only home visits [71, 72].

Table 10. CHWs and health promotion and disease prevention: pediatric immunization interventions

Author, Year Study Design Population Setting Sample Size Quality	Intensity of CHW Intervention	Study Groups	Results
Rask et al.,, 2001; [69] LeBaron et al., 2004 [70] RCT Pediatric Immunizations		G1: Autodial – automated telephone call delivered recorded message from health department medical staff; if no number or nonworking – then postcard to remind families 7 calendar days before child was due to be immunized	Vaccine series completed per immunization registry after 22 months: No statistical difference between CHW and control groups
Children <12 months in a county public health clinic in metropolitan Atlanta, Georgia N: 3,050 Good	Moderate	G2: Outreach – Following standardized protocol, outreach worker contacted patient within 1 week and made reminder call before appointment; if child still not up to date, monthly home visits attempted G3: Combination of G1 and G2 G4: Normal clinic procedure (control)	
Barnes et al., 1999 [68] RCT Pediatric Immunizations Low-income children in Manhattan, New York N: 434	Moderate	G1: Basic immunization education and referral. During subsequent contacts (home visits or telephone calls) throughout the remainder of followup, families were reminded of upcoming vaccinations and were recontacted to ensure that requisite vaccines were received. Contact with the clinic or escort to appointments provided if a family required support or assistance to obtain immunization services.	Up-to-date on immunizations after 6 months: G1: 75% G2: 54% ($P = 0.03$) Late for immunization: G1: 18% G2: 38% ($P < 0.05$)
Fair		G2: Informed of their child's immunization status at the enrollment visit by the control group interviewer and were instructed to reschedule the missed appointment.	
Barnes-Boyd et al., 2001 [71] Prospective Cohort Pediatric Immunizations Low-income inner-city African-American women and infants in Chicago, Illinois N: 1,922 Poor	High	G1: Monthly home visits over 1 year; visits at prenatal, 1, 6, and 12 months teamed with a nurse. G2: Historic controls with nurse home visits.	Percent fully immunized at12 months: G1: 77% G2: 63% ($P < 0.001$)

CHW, community health worker; G, group; N, number; RCT, randomized controlled trial.

Monthly home visits started prenatally and ended at 1 year [71, 72]. We rated this study poor because of high potential for secular trends, given the time difference between the two groups, and for other confounding problems [71, 72].

Overview of results. These three studies [68-72] evaluated the impact of CHWs on vaccine series completion rates and showed different CHW effectiveness. The good-quality study found no difference between groups receiving the CHW intervention and the control group [69, 70]. In contrast, the fair-quality study demonstrated that children in the CHW group were more up-to- date and less likely to be late for their immunizations than the controls [68] The control group for this study received more intervention directed at improving immunization rates, which would diminish the apparent effectiveness of the CHW. This study was more intensive than either of the other two projects (regular home visits or telephone calls over 6 months to ensure that requisite vaccines were received); this factor may have produced the difference in effectiveness between studies. REACH-Futures [71, 72] also found that the CHW-intervention group had a higher proportion of fully immunized participants at 12 months than did the historic controls who had received a nurse-only home visit.

Knowledge. No study reported outcomes for improved knowledge of pediatric immunization.

Behavior. No study reported outcomes for behavior changes.

Satisfaction. No study reported outcomes for satisfaction.

Health outcomes. All three studies evaluated immunization rates. The good-quality trial evaluated vaccine series completion rate from an immunization registry and found no difference between the CHW and control groups [69, 70]. The fair-quality trial found that children in the CHW arm were more up-to-date on immunizations than in the control arm (75 percent versus 54 percent, $P = 0.03$) and that fewer children were late for immunizations (18 percent versus 38 percent, $P < 0.5$) [68]. The poor-quality study evaluated vaccine series completion rates at 12 months and found that a higher proportion of children receiving the CHW and nurse home visits were up-to-date than historical controls ($P < 0.001$) [71, 72].

Health care utilization. No study reported outcomes for health care utilization.

Health promotion and disease prevention: health promotion – Latina health. *Study characteristics.* Two RCTs, one fair [66] and one poor quality [64, 65], examined outcomes of CHW interventions in comparison with mailings for health promotion in Latinas (Table 11). The fair- quality study used a moderate-intensity CHW intervention in uninsured Hispanic women age 40 years and older living at the US-Mexico border (Agua Prieta, Sonora, Mexico, and Douglas, Arizona, United States) with the aim of increasing return to clinic for an annual preventive examination [66]. It compared a group receiving CHW home visits in addition to reminder postcards with a group getting reminder postcards alone.

The poor-quality study, Secretos de la Buena Vida, used a high-intensity CHW model in the same target population living in San Diego County, California [64, 65]. It evaluated the effectiveness of weekly CHW home visits and telephone calls in addition to tailored print materials against that of tailored materials alone or off-the-shelf materials for changing dietary behavior. We rated this a poor-quality study because of a high potential for selection bias, measurement bias, and confounding [64, 65].

Overview of results. The fair study found that a moderate-intensity CHW intervention was more effective than a reminder postcard in increasing preventive exam appointments [66]. The poor-quality study demonstrated that a high-intensity CHW intervention group was different from those receiving weekly tailored dietary printed material in terms of dietary intake immediately post-intervention. This difference was no longer apparent after 6 months, although all three groups improved [64, 65].

Table 11. CHWs and health promotion and disease prevention: Latina health promotion interventions

Author, Year Study Design Population Setting Sample Size Quality	Intensity of CHW Intervention	Study Groups	Results
Hunter et al., 2004 [66] RCT Annual preventive exams Uninsured Hispanic women, aged 40 and older, living at the US-Mexico border N: 103 Fair	Moderate	G1: Received postcards in the mail 2 weeks before the month their annual exams were due, printed in language used to complete original questionnaire G2: Received G1 intervention and were visited by a promotora 2 weeks after the postcard had been mailed. Promotora facilitated appointment scheduling and contacted them to facilitate rescheduling if appointment was missed.	Return to clinic for a second comprehensive annual exam: G1: 48% (n = 24) G2: 65% (n = 33) RR, 1.35; 95% CI, 0.95-1.92
Elder et al., 2006; [65] Elder et al., 2005 [64] RCT: Secretos de La Buena Vida Dietary behavior, changes Latinas in San Diego County, California N: 357 Poor	High	G1: CHW home visits and/or telephone calls + tailored print materials G2: 12 weekly tailored newsletters and homework G3: 12 weekly off-the-shelf dietary printed material	Total fat gm, total fiber gm (Nutrition Data System 24-hour dietary recall interview) (validated): No significant difference between groups at 6 and 12 months postintervention

CHW, community health worker; CI, confidence interval; G, group; N, number; RCT, randomized controlled trial; RR, risk ratio.

Knowledge. Neither study reported outcomes for improved knowledge of health promotion.

Behavior. The Secretos de la Buena Vida project examined behavioral changes [64, 65]. The CHW arm and the tailored print arm did not differ significantly at 6 and 12 months postintervention in dietary intake of fat or fiber, based on a validated measure for 24-hour diet recall.

Satisfaction. Neither study reported outcomes for satisfaction.

Health outcomes. Neither study reported outcomes for improved health.

Health care utilization. The fair-quality, moderate-intensity CHW study reported on the percentage of women returning to clinic for a second annual preventive examination [66]. The CHW arm had a higher percentage of women returning than the postcard-only arm (65 percent versus 48 percent; RR, 1.35; 95percent CI, 0.95-1.92), but the difference was not statistically significant.

Health promotion and disease prevention: disease prevention. *Study characteristics.* Six studies, five RCTs [16, 67, 105, 107, 118, 119, 127] and one prospective cohort study [117], examined outcomes of CHW interventions for disease prevention in underserved populations throughout the United States (Table 12). Two studies were both high intensity and fair quality; [16, 67, 127] two studies were moderate intensity, one fair [105] and one poor quality; [118, 119] and two studies were low intensity, one fair [117] and one poor quality [107]. Studies focused on a broad range of disorders, including cardiovascular disease prevention [105, 118, 119], diabetes prevention [16, 127]. HIV prevention [117], colorectal cancer prevention [107], and second-hand smoke exposure [67] Of the five RCTs, three were of fair quality [16, 67, 105, 127] and two were poor [107, 118, 119].

The Missouri study was a fair-quality RCT evaluating a high-intensity CHW intervention focused on diabetes prevention in a low-income, African-American female population [16, 127]. This study compared 3 months of weekly sessions, alternating between group and individual sessions, targeting stages of change to tailor dietary patterns, with a control group that received a book to read [16, 127]. The San Diego study was a fair-quality RCT evaluating a high-intensity CHW intervention focused on decreasing secondary tobacco smoke exposure in Latino neighborhoods in San Diego County, California [67]. The intervention consisted of six home and/or telephone visits by CHWs over 4 months using culturally tailored behavioral problem-solving techniques to reduce secondary tobacco smoke exposure; controls received no intervention [67]. The Seattle, Washington, study was a fair-quality RCT evaluating moderate-intensity CHW assistance with medical followup against verbal advice to see a medical provider in low-income neighborhood participants who were found to have elevated blood pressure [105].

The sole prospective cohort study, rated fair quality, evaluated the effectiveness of a low-intensity CHW intervention in HIV prevention by street outreach to at-risk community members in Louisiana compared with a control group in a neighborhood receiving no intervention [117].

The poor-quality Baltimore, Maryland, trial evaluated a moderate-intensity intervention consisting of a nurse practitioner and CHW team at a nonclinical site with exercise equipment; CHWs provided dietary, smoking cessation, and exercise counseling [118, 119]. This strategy was compared with "enhanced" primary care, in which the same risk-specific materials and information on local programs were given to the intervention group and results and recommendations were provided to the patients' primary care physicians. We rated it poor because of a high potential for measurement bias [118, 119]. The WATCH trial was a poor-quality RCT of low intensity conducted in rural, predominantly African-American churches in North Carolina [107]. This study had four arms: (1) control churches offered a health education session and speakers not related to study objectives; (2) CHW intervention, consisting of organization and presentation of at least three church-wide activities on educating and enhancing support for healthy lifestyle and colorectal cancer screening; (3) four personalized computer-tailored newsletters and four targeted videotapes focused on healthy lifestyle and colorectal screening mailed bimonthly to participants' homes; and (4) both the CHW and the videotape components [107].

Overview of results. These six disease prevention studies reported on outcomes of knowledge, behavior, health outcomes, and health care utilization. Overall, four studies found that a CHW intervention was more effective in achieving outcomes than the respective control group [16, 105, 117-119, 127]. Two fair-quality studies (the Missouri trial [16, 127] and the prospective cohort study [117]) reported improved knowledge of the respective diseases in the CHW intervention as compared to respective controls. Two fair-quality studies (the Missouri trial [16, 127] and the prospective cohort study [117]) and one poor-quality study (the Baltimore trial [118, 119]) demonstrated that moderate- and low-intensity CHW interventions were more effective than controls in changing health behaviors.

The two studies that targeted tobacco cessation found opposing results regarding CHW effectiveness [67, 118, 119]. The fair-quality study (San Diego trial [67]) found no difference in smoking cessation between a high-intensity CHW intervention group and a group receiving nothing based on validated radioimmunoassay (RIA) of children's hair for nicotine and cotinine. The poor- quality study (Baltimore trial [118, 119]) found a significant difference between a moderate-intensity CHW intervention and enhanced usual care; however, this outcome was based on self-report. The fair-quality Seattle trial measured health care utilization and demonstrated that a moderate- intensity CHW intervention increased medical followup compared with only verbal advice to seek medical care for elevated blood pressure [105].

Overall, most (four of the six) disease prevention studies demonstrated that various levels of CHW intervention intensity (low, moderate, or high) were more effective than the comparator, which ranged from nothing to enhanced usual clinical care, in changing a variety of outcomes.

Table 12. CHWs and health promotion and disease prevention: disease prevention interventions

Author, Year Study Design Population Setting Sample Size Quality	Intensity of CHW Intervention	Study Groups	Results
Auslander et al., 2002; [16] Williams et al., 2001 [127] RCT Diabetes prevention Low-income African-American women in a large city (unspecified) in Missouri N: 294 Fair	High	G1: 6 group sessions (approximately 6 to 8 participants per group) and 6 individual sessions targeting stages of change to tailor, dietary pattern with a peer educator, meeting weekly over a 3-month period G2: A book (control)	Food Frequency Questionnaire – Validated: Intervention was effective in reducing fat intake, as measured by percentage of calories from total fat (baseline/6 months): G2: 36.0/34.5 G1: 35.9/32.3 ($P < 0.05$) BMI: No significant difference between groups Knowledge of Label Reading Questionnaire (unvalidated) baseline/6 months: G2: 5.4/5.7 G1: 5.5/6.3 ($P > 0.0001$)
Conway, 2004 [67] RCT Secondary tobacco smoke Latino neighborhoods in San Diego County, California N: 143 Fair	High	G1: Culturally relevant home and telephone visits on problem-solving techniques to reduce ETS exposure G2: No intervention (control)	RIA of child's hair for nicotine and cotinine (validated): No significant difference between groups
Krieger, 1999 [105] RCT Hypertension Low-income neighborhoods in Seattle, Washington N: 421 Fair	Moderate	G1: CHW assistance with medical followup related to a date when blood pressure was determined to be elevated G2: Advice to see medical provider, list of public and community clinics	Self-report of completed followup appointment within 90 days (validated by medical provider report): G1: 65.1% G2: 46.7% ($P = 0.001$)
Wendell, 2003 [117] Prospective cohort study	Low	G1: Discussions with community members during which they assessed the client's needs,	Condom use (intervention vs. comparison): OR, 1.37 (95% CI, 1.20 to 1.5;

Author, Year Study Design Population Setting Sample Size Quality	Intensity of CHW Intervention	Study Groups	Results
HIV prevention At-risk neighborhoods in Louisiana N: 6,547 Fair		imparted a risk- or harm-reduction message, answered questions, made referrals, and negotiated and reinforced behavior change G2: No intervention (control)	$P < 0.001$)
Becker et al., 2005; [118]Cene et al., 2008 [119] RCT Cardiovascular disease prevention Baltimore, Maryland N: 267 Poor	Moderate	G1: EPC- received risk-specific materials (same as intervention group), PCP received results and recommendations, sent info on local programs (e.g., YMCA) G2: CBC - received care in 1 nonclinical site in the community from a NP and CHW. CHW provided dietary counseling, smoking cessation, and exercise counseling lasting 30 minutes.	Smoking cessation (self-report): G1: 7% reduction G2: 16.2% reduction ($P < 0.001$)
Campbell, 2004 [107] RCT Colorectal cancer screening African-American rural churches in North Carolina NR (12 churches; completers/dropouts of individual participants from each church not reported) Poor	Low	G1: Control churches were offered health education sessions and speakers on topics of their choice not directly related to study objectives G2: Organize and conduct at least 3 church-wide activities on spreading info and enhancing support for healthy lifestyle and CRC screening (LHA) G3: 4 personalized computer-tailored newsletters and 4 targeted videotapes corresponding to the same behaviors mailed to participants' homes bimonthly for first 6 months after baseline data collection; 4th mailing was 9 months baseline G4: LHA + targeted print and videotape	Dietary change—daily fruit and vegetable servings (baseline/followup): G1: 3.3/3.4 G2: 3.5/3.5 G3: 3.3/3.9 G4: 3.4/3.7 No significant change across arms for LHA interventions Physical activity—recreational (moderate-vigorous) activity MET hours/week, M (SE) (baseline/followup): G1: 9.3(0.88)/8.4(0.69) G2: 10.5(0.9)/10.6(0.70) G3: 9.5(0.80)/10.9(0.61) G4: 9.7(0.76)/9.7(0.60) No significant change across arms for LHA interventions

BMI, body mass index; CBC, community-based care; CHW, community health worker; CI, confidence interval; EPC, enhanced primary care; ETS, environmental tobacco smoke; LHA, lay health advisor; MET, metabolic equivalent; N, number; NP, nurse practitioner; OR, odds ratio; PCP, primary care physician; RCT, randomized controlled trial; RIA, radioimmunoassay; SE, standard error; YMCA, Young Men's Christian Association.

Knowledge. Two fair-quality studies [16, 117, 127] reported outcomes for improved knowledge of the respective diseases. The Missouri study [16, 127] found that participants in the high-intensity, diabetes-oriented CHW intervention, compared with a control group receiving a book to read, had an improved knowledge of label reading as assessed by an unvalidated questionnaire ($P < 0.0001$); this improvement remained statistically significant at 6-month followup. The prospective cohort study [117] demonstrated that a low-intensity CHW street outreach program was effective at increasing knowledge of where to obtain free condoms as determined by an unvalidated questionnaire (90 percent versus 74 percent, odds ratio [OR], 3.2, $P = 0.001$).

Behavior. Five RCTs, three fair [16, 67, 105, 127] and two poor quality [107, 118, 119], examined a variety of behavioral changes. Three demonstrated CHW effectiveness [16, 105, 118, 119, 127] and two [67, 107] showed no difference compared with their respective controls. The Missouri trial on diabetes prevention evaluated dietary change following high-intensity, CHW-led group and individual sessions; [16, 127] it found a reduction in fat intake with a validated food frequency questionnaire compared with intake in a control group ($P < 0.0001$). The San Diego trial, a high-intensity CHW intervention of home and telephone visits to reduce second-hand tobacco smoke exposure to children, found no difference from baseline by self-report or validated RIA of children's hair for nicotine and cotinine [67]. In contrast, the Baltimore trial evaluated a CHW intervention and found a difference in self-reported smoking cessation as compared to a standard of care group (16.2 percent reduction versus 7.0 percent, $P < 0.001$) [118, 119]. Both groups reported less smoking, confirmed by measures of hair cotinine. The North Carolina trial did not show a difference in either fruit and vegetable intake or increased physical activity between intervention and control groups [107] The prospective cohort low-intensity study targeting HIV prevention demonstrated an increase in condom use reported in the intervention group (OR, 1.37; 95 percent CI, 1.20-1.56) [117].

Satisfaction. No study for health promotion evaluated outcomes focused on satisfaction.

Health outcomes. The Missouri trial found no difference within or between arms when comparing the high-intensity CHW intervention and the control group in terms of body weight and body mass index (BMI) at baseline (BMI 35.7 versus 35.3) and after 6 months (BMI 35.7 versus 35.4) [16, 127].

Health care utilization. The Seattle trial evaluated self-reported medical provider followup within 90 days of determined elevated blood pressure [105]. It demonstrated a higher rate of completed medical followup in the CHW group than in the control group (65.1 percent versus 46.7 percent, $P = 0.001$). The number needed to treat in order to bring 1 person to medical care was 5 (95 CI, 3-13) [105].

Outcomes for Injury Prevention

Injury prevention: home safety. *Study characteristics.* One fair-quality RCT [101] and one poor-quality RCT randomized at the community level (called the Safe Block Project) [102] assessed the effect of low-intensity CHW interventions on injury prevention in homes, either for children [101] or for all ages [102]. Both studies involved CHW home visits. The fair-quality RCT consisted of assessment of safety hazards and recommendations for appropriate products and practices compared with safety counseling in a pediatric clinic [101]. The poor-quality RCT also included direct implementation of several safety features into homes compared with no intervention in control households; we rated this trial poor because of its high potential for measurement bias and not masking those who assessed outcomes [102].

Overview of results. The fair-quality RCT showed no benefit to CHW intervention [101], but the poor-quality trial had mixed results [102] (Table 13.). Significant benefit was seen for household features that did not require participants to change behaviors (e.g., continued presence of a smoke detector, as installed in intervention homes); conversely, no benefit was observed for other household features that did require behavior change (e.g., maintaining a working light bulb in stairways).

Table 13. CHW injury prevention interventions and home safety

Author, Year Study Design Population Setting Sample Size Quality	Intensity of CHW Intervention	Study Groups	Results
Gielen et al., 2002 [101] Parents and infants 6 months or younger in large urban teaching hospital pediatric clinic Baltimore, Maryland N: 187 Fair	Moderate	G1: Safety counseling and referral by pediatrician to children's safety center G2: Standard care plus offer of CHW home visit; assessed injury hazards; made recommendations about appropriate safety products and practices; referred families to the children's safety center; 1 visit between 6 and 9 months	No significant difference between groups in home safety practices: Hot water temperature controlled: Pre/Post G1: 39%/47%; G2: 39%/47% Working smoke alarm: Pre/Post G1: 92%/84%; G2: 92%/81% Safety gates used: Pre (planned use)/Post (actual use) G1: 84%/23%; G2: 84%/27% Poisons latched/locked: Pre/Post G1: 26%/12%; G2: 26%/10% Ipecac present: Pre/Post G1: 12%/27%; G2: 12%/31%
Schwarz et al., 1993 [102] (Safe Block Study) Inner city residents in neighborhoods with high injury rates Philadelphia, Pennsylvania N: 2,722 Poor	Moderate	G1: Safety inspections, home modifications and education; myriad safety devices (e.g., smoke detectors, ipecac, emergency telephone numbers, light bulbs) G2: Control (details NR)	G1 more likely than G2 to retain intervention modifications such as presence of ipecac ($P < 0.001$), hot water temperature control ($P < 0.001$) No difference between groups for adequate lighting at stairs

CHW, community health worker; G, group; N, number.

Knowledge. Neither study assessed knowledge-related outcomes.

Behavior. In the fair-quality RCT [101], groups did not differ significantly in maintaining adequate stairway lighting (83.1 percent versus 80.1 percent; adjusted odds ratio [AOR], 0.90; 95 percent CI, 0.69-1.16) or in following any of the home safety practices assessed. Hot water temperature control and presence of ipecac increased from baseline in both groups, but presence of a working smoke alarm, use of safety gates on stairs, and latching or locking of poisons declined from baseline. In the poor-quality trial [102], following the CHW intervention a significantly higher proportion of households continued to have ipecac (which was recommended at the time of the study for households with young children) (81.0 percent versus 9.8 percent; AOR, 0.04; 95 percent CI, 0.02 to 0.07) and smoke detectors (96.0 percent versus 77 percent; AOR, 0.14; 95 percent CI, 0.09 to 0.20) than did controls. These interventions were provided by the CHWs and required no behavior change by participants. In contrast, intervention households were actually less likely than control households to have retained hot water temperature controls (63.2 percent versus 73.2 percent; AOR, 1.73; 95 percent CI, 1.39 to 2.15).

Satisfaction. Neither study assessed satisfaction.

Health outcomes. Neither study assessed direct health outcomes.

Health care utilization. Neither study assessed health care utilization.

Injury prevention: workplace safety. *Study characteristics.* One prospective cohort study, rated poor quality for high potential for selection and measurement bias and lack of description of baseline characteristics, examined the effect of a low-intensity CHW intervention for migrant farm workers to prevent work-related eye injury. The CHW intervention involved distribution of protective eyewear either with or without specific training provided by the CHWs; it was compared to distribution of eye protection not involving CHWs. Outcomes were assessed during the same growing season in parts of the Midwest.

Overview of results. The CHW intervention increased the likelihood of protective eyewear use, particularly when coupled with CHW-led training (Table 14) [126].

Knowledge. Knowledge was not assessed.

Behavior. The presence of any CHW component related to receiving protective eyewear was significantly associated with increased self-report of continued use of the eyewear on a 5-point Likert scale compared with having received the eyewear without CHW involvement (difference in average change in Likert scale value 0.6452, $P < 0.01$). Incorporation of CHW-led training was associated with greater self-reported eyewear use compared with CHW eyewear distribution alone (difference in average change 0.7663, $P < 0.01$) and with no CHW involvement (difference in average change 0.5241, $P = 0.03$). Observed use of eyewear increased in all groups during the study period (CHW trained 1.1 to 36 percent; CHW distributed 0 to 5.2 percent; no CHW 0 to 14 percent, *P*-value not reported).

Satisfaction. Satisfaction was not assessed.

Health outcomes. Although the investigators measured the incidence of pterygium, they did not compare groups on this variable and in fact reported it as only inadequately identified.

Health care utilization. No measure of health care utilization was reported.

Table 14. CHW injury prevention interventions and workplace safety

Author, Year Study Design Population Setting Sample Size Quality	Intensity of CHW Intervention	Study Groups	Results
Forst et al., 2004 [126] Latino migrant and seasonal farm workers Southeast Michigan and northeast Illinois N: 786 Poor	Low intensity	G1: CHW distributed protective eyewear, conducted at least 1 each individual and group training sessions G2: CHW distributed eyewear, did not provide training G3: No CHW component	G1 were more likely to increase use of protective eyewear compared with G2 ($P< 0.0001$) and with G3 ($P= 0.03$) Any CHW intervention increased likelihood of protective eyewear use vs. no CHW ($P= 0.0004$)

CHW, community health worker; G, group; N, number.

Outcomes for Maternal and Child Health

Maternal and child health: overview. We identified 15 studies that met inclusion criteria and involved maternal or child health outcomes (or both). All the studies utilized high-intensity interventions, usually involving some series of home visits. All but 1 study were rated either fair (8 studies) or poor (6 studies). The 1 good-quality study found no significant differences associated with interventions employing CHWs. Among the other studies, results were mixed, some showing benefit of CHW interventions and some showing no effect attributable to CHWs. This distribution was found in both fair- and poor-quality studies. Significant associations were most commonly found for existing conditions (e.g., phenylketonuria [PKU] or failure to thrive) rather than primary prevention and in the area of health care utilization (e.g., immunization rates) and behavior (e.g., parenting measures).

Maternal and child health: prenatal care and perinatal outcomes. *Study characteristics.* Six studies assessed prenatal care and perinatal outcomes associated with CHWs [71, 72, 77, 79, 83, 86, 87]. Of these, three were rated fair quality: one RCT involving prenatal care in Cleveland79 and two cohort studies (one on the Resource Mothers Program for Maternal PKU [83] and one evaluating REACH-Futures [72]). The remaining three studies, rated poor, included one RCT on promotion of breastfeeding in African-American mothers in Baltimore [77], rated poor for high attrition and lack of specific or validated outcome measures; one cohort study (the Baby Love Maternal Outreach Worker study [31, 32]), rated poor for high attrition, high potential for selection bias and confounding, and lack of specific or validated outcome measures; and a second study on REACH-Futures [71] rated poor for high potential for secular trend and other confounding.

Most studies focused on interventions for low-income families, usually from racial or ethnic minority groups. Most CHW interventions involved home visits. The Resource Mothers Program for Maternal PKU [83] involved coaching in activities of daily living unique to mothers with PKU infants including meal planning and medical recommendations concerning pregnancy. The Maternal Outreach Worker program also provided direct assistance to families for obtaining benefits and services [86, 87].

Studies generally compared outcomes for families receiving CHW interventions with outcomes for those receiving usual clinical care (Table 15). The Baltimore breastfeeding study compared CHW intervention with video and other literature and against both interventions combined; [77] the Resource Mothers Program [83] used as controls mothers who had completed pregnancy in the 5 years before the start of the program; and REACH-Futures [71, 72] used historic controls of nurse home visits. Outcomes were typically assessed months to years after the interventions.

Overview of results. Improvements over usual care were demonstrated to be associated with CHWs in breastfeeding [77], maternal control of PKU [83], and prenatal care [86, 87]. However, birth outcomes in mothers with PKU [83], low birth weight incidence [86, 87], continuation of breastfeeding [77], and overall presence of infant health problems [71] were not significantly improved by use of CHWs compared with usual care [77, 83, 86, 87] or with health professional intervention [71].

Knowledge. No study measured knowledge-related outcomes.

Behavior. No study assessed behavior change.

Health outcomes. Peer CHW counseling in the Baltimore study was associated with greater initiation of breastfeeding than standard care (OR, 3.84; 95 percent CI, 1.44-10.21), but the statistically significant difference between groups in the proportion of participants still breastfeeding by 7 to 10 days disappeared [77]. For the Resource Mothers Program [83], mothers receiving the CHW intervention needed less time to reach metabolic control (blood phenylalanine level consistently below 10 mg/dL) than those who had not received the intervention (8.5 weeks versus 16 weeks, $P < 0.05$). The head circumference of infants born to participating mothers did not differ significantly between cohorts (mean Z-score of head circumference: intervention -0.56; 95 percent CI, -0.88 - -0.24 versus control -1.4; 95 percent CI, -1.56 - -1.2; $P = 0.08$). The Maternal Outreach Workers program demonstrated a trend toward lower incidence of adequate prenatal care for African-American women receiving CHW intervention than for controls (significance not reported); [86, 87] neither the observed nor the expected incidences of low birth weight or very low birth weight infants differed significantly. REACH-Futures found no difference between CHW intervention and controls in incidence of neonatal or postneonatal infant health problems [71].

Health care utilization. The Cleveland study showed a significant increase in the ratio of actual to expected numbers of prenatal visits for women receiving CHW intervention ($P = 0.029$); [79] the investigators did not compare the intervention findings to those from women in the control group.

Table 15. CHW maternal and child interventions and prenatal care and perinatal outcomes

Author, Year Study Design Population Setting Sample Size Quality	Intensity of CHW Intervention	Study Groups	Results
Graham et al., 1992 [79] RCT Pregnant inner-city African-American women Cleveland, Ohio N: 145 Fair	High	G1: Home visits with psychosocial support and encouragement, education, link to community resources, information on health risks; 4 visits of 1 hour each at 2-4 week intervals G2: Routine prenatal obstetric care (control)	No statistically significant difference between groups in incidence of low birth weight: 12.9% intervention, 7.5% controls ($P = 0.51$)
Nacion et al., 2000 [72] Cohort REACH-Futures Low-income inner-city African-American pregnant women and infants Chicago, Illinois N: 213 Fair	High	G1: Home visits by CHW G2: Home visits by nurse (historic control)	G1 more likely than G2 to receive problem-solving services ($P < 0.01$) and to have problems identified in women's health ($P = 0.01$), well-child health care deficits ($P = 0.02$), parenting ($P = 0.02$), and socioeconomic issues ($P < 0.01$) G1 less likely than G2 to receive emotional support services ($P < 0.01$), to have referrals placed for women's health ($P = 0.01$), well-woman ($P = 0.02$), emotional/interpersonal ($P < 0.01$), parental support ($P < 0.01$), or for socioeconomic issues ($P < 0.01$)

Author, Year Study Design Population Setting Sample Size Quality	Intensity of CHW Intervention	Study Groups	Results
St. James et al., 1999 [83] Cohort Mothers with PKU New England N: 69 Fair	High	G1: Historic control; women who completed pregnancy in the 5 years prior to project onset G2: Resource mothers	Metabolic control achieved in 8.5 weeks for G2 vs. 16 weeks for G1 ($P < 0.05$) Infant mental scale on Bayley Developmental Quotient was 108 for G2 vs.95 for G1 ($P < 0.05$) No difference in head circumference at birth($P = 0.08$)
Barnes-Boyd et al., 2001 [71] Cohort REACH-Futures Low-income inner-city African-American pregnant women and infants Chicago, Illinois N: 1,922 Poor	High	G1: Monthly home visits over 1 year; visits at prenatal, 1, 6, and 12 months teamed with nurse G2: Historic controls with nurse home visits	Proportion fully immunized at 12 months:CHW 77%, nurse 63% ($P < 0.001$) No significant difference between groups in presence of neonatal or postneonatal health problems (27% CHW vs. 25% nurse)
Caulfield et al., 1998[77] RCT African-American women receiving prenatal care Baltimore, Maryland N: 548 Poor	High	G1: Standard WIC services only G2: WIC plus video and literature G3: WIC plus peer counseling G4: WIC plus peer counseling plus video and literature	Initiation of breastfeeding: G1: 26% (referent) G2: 50% (OR, 1.36; 95% CI, 0.52-3.54) G3: 62% (OR, 3.84; 95% CI, 1.44-10.21) G4: 52% (OR, 1.92; 95% CI, 0.78-4.76) Breastfeeding at 7-10 days: G1: 14% (referent) G2: 30% (OR, 0.79; 95% CI, 0.25-2.52) G3: 38% (OR, 1.11; 95% CI, 0.34-3.61) G4: 38% (OR, 1.52; 95% CI, 0.50-4.59)
Tessaro et al., 1997 [86, 87] Cohort Maternal Outreach Workers Medicaid-eligible pregnant women with 1 or more pregnancy risk factors North Carolina N: 705 Poor	High	G1: CHW intervention G2: Matched controls, not otherwise defined	Maternal depression score increased by 2.1 in G1 vs. 5.1 in G2 ($P = 0.01$) Prenatal care, African Americans: G1: 60.7% adequate, 32.6% intermediate, 6.7% inadequate G2: 63.8% adequate, 31.5% intermediate, 4.7% inadequate Prenatal care, Whites: G1: 77.4% adequate, 19.7% intermediate, 2.9% inadequate G2: 75.1% adequate, 22.8% intermediate, 2.1% inadequate No difference between groups in maternal self-esteem ($P = 0.19$) or perceived stress ($P = 0.75$) No difference in observed vs. expected incidence of low birth weight or very low birth weight: African Americans -13 ($P = 0.12$), Whites +1 ($P = 0.58$)

CHW, community health worker; PKU, phenylketonuria; WIC, Special Supplemental Nutrition Program for Women, Infants, and Children.

Other. The fair-quality analysis from REACH-Futures found that CHW home visits were more likely than nurse home visits to include identification of problems in women's health ($P = 0.01$), deficits in well-child care ($P = 0.02$), parenting issues ($P = 0.02$), and socioeconomic issues ($P < 0.01$) and that participants were more likely to receive problem-solving services ($P < 0.01$) [72]. However, CHWs were less likely than nurses to provide emotional support services ($P < 0.01$) or to place referrals for women's health ($P = 0.01$), well-woman care ($P = 0.02$), emotional/interpersonal support ($P < 0.01$), parental support ($P < 0.01$), or socioeconomic issues ($P < 0.01$).

Maternal and child health: Child development. *Study characteristics.* Four studies considered the impact of CHWs on child development (Table 16). Three were rated fair quality and one poor quality; all used high-intensity interventions. One RCT focused on children with nonorganic failure to thrive in Baltimore, Maryland; [75, 76] another RCT examined the Home Visitation 2000 program in Denver, Colorado; [80-82] and a cohort study involved the Resource Mothers Program for Maternal PKU in New England [83]. The RCT assessing the Hawaii Healthy Start Program [78, 128] was rated poor for high potential for site-specific bias.

Overview of results. Variation in timing and specific outcomes among studies precludes much summarization of results. Two of the studies demonstrated some significant benefit of CHW intervention over usual care; the other two showed no significant difference between CHW intervention and controls. The failure-to-thrive study demonstrated that the CHW home visiting program was effective in mitigating declines in cognitive and motor development, but not language, if implemented during the first year of life (Table 16) [75, 76]. The PKU Resource Mothers Program study found higher mental development for infants born to mothers who participated than for those born to historic controls [83] By contrast, the Home Visitation 2000 trial showed more improvement in language development with nurse visits rather than CHWs [80-82], and the Hawaii trial found no difference in mental or psychomotor development between children receiving CHW intervention and controls.

Knowledge. No study assessed knowledge about child development issues.

Behavior. No study included health behaviors in the outcomes measured.

Satisfaction. No study considered satisfaction outcomes.

Health outcomes. All four studies examined various health outcomes. In the Baltimore, Maryland, failure-to-thrive study, the decline in cognitive development over 1 year as measured by the Bayley Scales of Infant Development was less severe for the home intervention group than for the clinic-only group ($P = 0.02$) for children recruited during infancy. Groups of children recruited at older ages did not differ using the Battelle Developmental Inventory, although all groups demonstrated some degree of decline in cognitive function. Whether this decline was attributable to failure to thrive or to some other factor was not assessed in the study. Children in the intervention group showed less severe decline in receptive and expressive language than did age-matched controls ($P = 0.05$), but all groups experienced relative declines in language over the course of the study. All groups showed significant improvements in weight for age, weight for height, and height for age, but the groups did not differ significantly.

The Home Visitation 2000 study in Denver, Colorado, found slightly greater improvement over controls with nurse home visits than with CHW visits for the Preschool Language Scales at 21 months and the Mental Development Index at 24 months [80-82].

Infants in the intervention cohort of the Resource Mothers Program in New England had higher mean Bayley Developmental Quotient (mental scale) values than those in the control cohort (108 versus 95) at 12 months of age ($P < 0.05$) [83].

At 2 years postintervention, children in the Hawaii Healthy Start Program [78, 128] who received CHW intervention had a mean Bayley Mental Development Index score of 90.0 versus 89.2 for controls (*P* = 0.60) and a Psychomotor Development Index score of 92.1 versus 90.4 for controls (*P* = 0.12).

Table 16. CHW maternal and child interventions and child development

Author, Year Population Setting Sample Size Quality	Intensity of CHW Intervention	Study Groups	Results
Black et al., 1995; [75] Hutcheson et al., 1997 [76] Low-income urban children with nonorganic failure to thrive Baltimore, Maryland N: 130 Fair	High	G1: Weekly CHW home visits with community health nurse supervision for 1 year, addressing various child health and development needs, nutrition intervention, and concerns raised by mothers G2: Clinic-based multidisciplinary services; no CHW intervention	Smaller postintervention decline in cognitive and motor development for G1 vs. G2 only for children recruited in infancy Bayley cognitive development (SD): G1: 96.9 (SD 15.8) to 89.3 (17.4) G2: 96.2 (12.1) to 86.1 (18.7) Bayley motor development: G1: 91.1 (18.7) to 92.0 (14.6) G2: 95.3 (17.7) to 91.5 (18.7) (*P*= 0.02) No significant differences between groups for language development
Korfmacher et al., 1999; [81] Olds et al., 2002; [80] Olds et al., 2004 [82] Home Visitation 2000 Medicaid-eligible pregnant women Denver, Colorado N: 735 Fair	High	G1: Developmental screening plus intensive home visitation: promoting healthy behaviors, competent child care, pregnancy planning, education, employment; linking to social and health services; promoting healthy family/friend relationships; variable frequency from weekly to monthly up to 24 months of age G2: Developmental screening plus nurse home visits G3: Developmental screening and referrals	Preschool Language Scales at 21months (G3 mean 99.49): G1 vs. G3 + 0.40 (95% CI, -1.94 to +2.74) G2 vs. G3 + 1.73 (95% CI, -0.64 to +4.11) Mental Development Index at 24 months (G3 mean 89.38): G1 vs. G3 + 0.07 (95% CI, -2.39 to +2.53) G2 vs. G3 + 0.75 (95% CI, -1.77 to +3.28)
St. James et al., 1999 [83] Mothers with PKU (PKU Resource Mothers Program) New England N: 69 Fair	High	G1: Historic control; women who completed pregnancy in the 5 years before project onset G2: Resource mothers	Infant mental scale on Bayley Developmental Quotient was G1: 95 G2: 108 (*P* < 0.05)
Duggan et al., 1999; [128] Duggan et al., 2000 [78] Families at high risk for child maltreatment Oahu, Hawaii N: 730 Poor	High	G1: Home visiting with individualized service plans, child developmental screenings, and mother-child interaction assessments; family support plan within 45 days of initial visit, reviewed every 6 months, revised annually; periodic screening for developmental delays, observational assessment of parent-child interaction and home environment; ensure existence of medical home, link to other needed resources G2: Control (details NR)	All outcome measures at 2 years postintervention Bayley Scales of Infant Development – Mental Development Index: G1: 90.0 G2: 89.2 (*P* = 0.60) Psychomotor Development Index: G1: 92.1 G2: 90.4 (*P* = 0.12)

CHW, community health workers; CI, confidence interval; G, group; PKU, phenylketonuria; SD, standard deviation.

Health care utilization. No study assessed health care utilization.

Maternal and child health: Environment conducive to child well-being. *Study characteristics.* Factors contributing to an environment conducive to the health and well-being of children were assessed directly in 10 studies; 6 rated as fair quality and 4 as poor quality. The five fair-quality RCTs covered the following populations and interventions: smokers in San Diego; [67] low-income urban children with nonorganic failure to thrive; [75, 76] the Parent to Parent Network for mothers of children with chronic conditions; [85] a trial targeting children in New York with missed immunization visits; [68] a trial involving drug-using mothers in Maryland; [84] and the Home Visitation 2000 RCT [80-82]. Finally, of the four poor-quality studies, two RCTs (both involving the Child-Parent Enrichment Project, or CPEP [73, 74]) were rated poor for lack of relevant outcome measures; the Hawaii Healthy Start Program [78, 128] was rated poor for high potential for site-specific bias; and on the REACH-Futures trial [71] was rated poor because of high potential for secular trend and for other confounding.

Overview of results. The variety of outcomes assessed by the studies precludes much summary of results. Of the 10 studies in this category, only 4 reported significantly beneficial outcomes for CHWs over usual care.

The New York study [68] and REACH-Futures trial [71] did find CHW-associated improvements in immunization status. Home Visitation 2000 showed greater improvement with nurse than with CHW interventions for mother-infant interaction, home environment, and tobacco smoke exposure [80-82]. The Hawaii study found that CHW intervention significantly increased appropriate parental coping and discipline methods and decreased injuries from partner-related violence [78, 128].

As to the remaining studies: the San Diego study found no significant impact by CHWs on exposure to environmental tobacco smoke among children of smokers [67]. The failure-to-thrive study found no effect of CHWs on outcomes related to home environment or parenting behavior [75, 76]. The Parent to Parent Network study showed no significant difference between intervention and control groups for maternal psychiatric well-being postintervention; [85] however, the results were potentially confounded by differences at baseline. No differences were found in the Maryland study [84] for maternal drug use or mother-child interaction. Other studies on substance abuse, child maltreatment, and improving psychiatric outcomes among caregivers of children with chronic diseases also did not report significant differences between study arms [74, 84]

Knowledge. No study assessed measures of knowledge.

Behavior. The failure-to-thrive study found no differences between groups for parent-child interaction behavior during feeding using a modified Parent Child Early Relational Assessment [75, 76]. It did show improved interactive communication with parents during feeding among children over time for all groups ($P < 0.001$), but no differences were apparent according to intervention status. Developmental appropriateness of the home environment, as assessed postintervention by the Home Observation for Measurement of the Environment Scales, was slightly higher for the CHW intervention group than for the clinic-only group (31.6 [SD 3.6] versus 29.3 [SD 4.2] for infants; 32.4 [SD 5.1] versus 30.3 [SD 5.7] for older children; $P = 0.05$ [significance not reported by age strata]). However, no baseline scores were reported for this measure to ascertain the true effect of CHWs.

Table 17. CHW maternal and child interventions and environment conducive to child health

Author, Year Study Design Population Setting Sample Size Quality	Intensity of CHW Intervention	Study Groups	Results
Barnes et al., 1999 [68] Low-income immigrant children from Dominican Republic NW Manhattan, New York N: 434 Fair	High	G1: Basic immunization education and referral; home visits with reminders of immunizations due, followup to ensure compliance G2: Information provided on child's missed immunizations, encouraged to reschedule missed appointments (control)	Immunizations up to date: G1: 75% G2: 54% ($P = 0.03$) Late for immunizations: G1: 18% G2: 38% ($P < 0.05$)
Conway et al., 2004 [67] Latino families with smokers and children between 1 and 9 years old San Diego County, California N: 143 Fair	High	G1: Home and telephone visits on problem-solving techniques to reduce environmental tobacco smoke exposure; 6 visits over 4 months G2: Participated in surveys but received no other intervention (control)	No difference between groups for parent report of child's tobacco exposure or child's hair nicotine or cotinine levels (no reduction in either group)
Black et al., 1995 [75]; Hutcheson et al., 1997 [76] Low-income urban children with nonorganic failure to thrive Baltimore, Maryland N: 130 Fair	High	G1: Weekly CHW home visits with community health nurse supervision for 1 year, addressing various child health and development needs, nutrition intervention, and concerns raised by mothers G2: Clinic-based multidisciplinary services; no CHW intervention	No significant differences between groups for parent-child interaction HOMES home environment scores not reported pre-intervention
Korfmacher et al., 1999; [81] Olds et al., 2002; [80] Olds et al., 2004 [82] (Home Visitation 2000) Medicaid-eligible pregnant women Denver, Colorado Fair N: 735	High	G1: Developmental screening plus intensive home visitation: promoting healthy behaviors, competent child care, pregnancy planning, education, employment; linking to social and health services; promoting healthy family/friend relationships; variable frequency from weekly to monthly up to 24 months of age G2: Developmental screening plus nurse home visits G3: Developmental screening and referrals (control)	Greater improvement in mother-infant interaction and home environment with intervention vs. controls for nursehome visits (least squares mean 1.32, $P \leq 0.05$) than for CHW visits (least squares mean 1.16, $P < 0.1$) Urine cotinine among smoking mothers reduced in all groups, more so for nurse intervention: CHW vs. control -76.19 ng/dL (95% CI, -302.21 to -149.82) Nurse vs. control -246.68 ng/dL (95% CI, -466.19 to -27.16; $P \leq 0.05$)

Table 17. (Continued)

Author, Year Study Design Population Setting Sample Size Quality	Intensity of CHW Intervention	Study Groups	Results
Schuler et al., 2000 [84] Women with known history of drug use plus their infants Unspecified inner city, Maryland N: 192 Fair	High	G1: 9 visits of 30 minutes each to enhance mothers' ability to manage self-identified problems by using existing services and family and social supports; modeling infant development behavior/activities G2: 3 monthly visits of 17 minutes each for tracking purposes only	No difference between groups in self-reported maternal drug use or in infant warmth on observed mother-child interactions 65% of intervention and 68% of controls reported alcohol use postintervention, 46% of intervention and 44% of controls reported cocaine and/or heroin use, 25% of intervention and 38% of controls reported marijuana use ($P \geq 0.1$)
Silver et al., 1997 [85] Inner-city, low-income, minority women with children who have a chronic disease Bronx or Lower Westchester, New York N: 365 Fair	High	G1: Intervention G2: Usual care (control)	Psychiatric Symptom Index scores higher at baseline in G1 than G2 ($P< 0.05$), but no difference between groups postintervention
Barnes-Boyd et al., 2001 [71] (REACH-Futures) Low-income inner-city African-American pregnant women and infants Chicago, Illinois N: 1,922 Poor	High	G1: Monthly home visits over 1 year; visits at prenatal, 1, 6, and 12 months teamed with nurse G2: Nurse home visits (historic controls)	Proportion fully immunized at 12 months: CHW 77%, nurse 63% ($P< 0.001$)
Barth et al., 1988 [73] Families referred for high risk of child maltreatment Contra Costa County, California N: 65 Poor	High	G1: Twice-monthly home visits over 6 months with links to other community resources G2: Usual care	Child Abuse Potential Inventory pre-vs. postintervention: G1: 116.33 (SD 47.75) to 88.54 (SD 53.09) G2: 103.50 (SD 43.26) to 92.44 (SD 51.44) ($P\geq0.05$ between groups)
Barth et al., 1991 [74] Families referred for high risk of child maltreatment Contra Costa County, California N: 240 Poor	High	G1: Home visits G2: Usual care	Increase in total child maltreatment-related reports and court actions: G1: +40 families to +65 total reports G2: +41 families to +74 total reports (no significance testing reported)
Duggan et al., 1999; [128] Duggan et al., 2000 [78]	High	G1: Home visiting with individualized service plans, child developmental screenings, and mother-child	All outcome measures at 2 years postintervention Reported frequent use of nonviolent discipline strategies:

Author, Year Study Design Population Setting Sample Size Quality	Intensity of CHW Intervention	Study Groups	Results
Families at high risk for child maltreatment Oahu, Hawaii N: 730 Poor		interaction assessments; family support plan within 45 days of initial visit, reviewed every 6 months, revised annually; periodic screening for developmental delays, observational assessment of parent-child interaction and home environment; ensure existence of medical home, links to other needed resources G2: Control (details NR)	G1: 39% G2: 34% ($P = 0.03$) Reported parenting-related stress: G1: 77.7% G2: 80.7% ($P = 0.08$) Parenting efficacy (Parenting Sense of Confidence Scale): G1: 76.1 G2: 74.1 ($P = 0.03$) Maternal life skills (Community Life Skills Scale): G1: 23.9 G2: 23.9 ($P = 0.84$) Maternal social support (Maternal Social Support Index): G1: 21.4 G2: 21.7 ($P = 0.48$) Maternal substance use: G1: 18% G2: 20% ($P = 0.55$) Maternal depressive symptoms: G1: 23% G2: 26% ($P = 0.49$) Poor, general maternal mental health: G1: 36% G2: 39% ($P = 0.43$) Home learning environment (Total Home Observation for Measurement of the Environment Scale): G1: 34.6 G2: 34.1 ($P = 0.47$) Mother-child interaction (Nursing Child Assessment Satellite Training scales): G1: Caregiver total 15.0, child total 7.2 G2: Caregiver total 14.6 ($P = 0.28$), child total 7.2 ($P = 0.83$) Partner-related violence in household resulting in injury: G1: 16% G2: 24% ($P = 0.03$) Confirmed Child Protective Services
			reports: G1: 2% G2: 3% ($P = 0.40$) Presence of primary care provider: G1: 91% G2: 86% ($P = 0.09$) Adequate number of well-child visits: G1: 60% G2: 55% ($P = 0.95$) Immunizations up to date: G1: 87% G2: 85% ($P = 0.45$)

CHW, community health worker; CI, confidence interval; G, group; N, number; ng/dL, nanograms/deciliter; SD, standard deviation.

In the Maryland study on substance-abusing mothers, self-reported postintervention substance use was similar for mothers receiving CHW interventions and for those in the control group (65 percent versus 68 percent for alcohol, 46 percent versus 44 percent for cocaine and/or heroin, and 25 percent versus 38 percent for marijuana; $P \geq 0.1$) [84].

The Hawaii study found that parents who received CHW intervention had a greater postintervention use of nonviolent discipline strategies (see Table 16), reported less parenting- related stress, and had higher parenting efficacy scores than those receiving usual care alone [78, 128].

Satisfaction. No study assessed satisfaction outcomes.

Health outcomes. Among children of smokers in the San Diego study [67], no reduction was seen in parental report of children's tobacco exposure or in nicotine or cotinine levels in children's hair for either CHW or control participants. The Parent to Parent Network demonstrated no difference between groups in postintervention Psychiatric Symptom Index scores (intervention 22.1 versus control 20.1) [85]. However, the baseline score for the intervention group was significantly higher than for the control group (24.1 versus 20.3, respectively; $P < 0.05$). Adjustment for this baseline difference revealed a greater degree of improvement in the intervention group than in controls, except for the depression subscale, which was improved in both groups. However, whether this reflected true improvement attributable to CHWs or was simply a regression to the mean could not be determined. The New York study showed that children receiving CHW intervention were more likely than control children to be current on their immunizations ($P = 0.03$) and less likely to have received immunizations behind schedule ($P < 0.05$) (Table 17) [68].

The Maryland study found infant warmth (on a 5-point scale) to be equal for those receiving CHW interventions and controls (2.5, SD 0.4 for both groups) [84].

Home Environment 2000 demonstrated more improvement over controls in mother-infant interaction and in home environment for nurse home visits (least squares mean 1.32, $P \leq 0.05$) than for CHW visits (least squares mean 1.16, $P < 0.1$) [80-82]. Among participating families with mothers who smoked, maternal urine cotinine was reduced in all groups; those receiving nurse home visits had a significantly greater degree of reduction than those receiving CHW visits (nurse versus control -246.68 ng/dL; 95 percent CI, -466.19 to -27.16); CHW versus control - 76.19 ng/dL; 95 percent CI, -302.21 to -149.82; $P \leq 0.05$).

The studies from Contra Costa, California, found no significant difference between groups on the Child Abuse Potential Inventory postintervention (Table 17); both groups showed improvement and no difference in reported cases of child maltreatment [73, 74].

The Hawaii study [78, 128] demonstrated no difference between groups for maternal life skills (Table 17), maternal social support, maternal substance use, maternal depressive symptoms, or incidence of poor general mental health among mothers at 2 years postintervention. Neither home learning environment nor parent-child interactions differed between groups at 2 years. The investigators did not report how each of these measures compared with baseline values. The study did show lower incidence of injuries attributable to partner-related violence among families receiving CHW intervention ($P = 0.03$), but no differences in reported or confirmed cases of child maltreatment.

Health care utilization. Children receiving CHW intervention in the Hawaii study were no more likely than those receiving usual care to have a primary care provider ($P = 0.09$) (Table 17), to have received the recommended number of well-child visits ($P = 0.95$), or to be current on immunization status ($P = 0.45$) [78, 128].

Outcomes for Cancer Screening

Cancer screening. *Study Characteristics.* A total of 15 studies (24 citations) examined outcomes of CHW interventions for improving breast, cervical, or colorectal cancer screening [15, 17-22, 59-63, 103, 104, 106-113, 116, 125]. Information on these studies is spread across multiple tables, depending on the specific focus: improving knowledge, changing behavior, breast self- examination, Pap smears, mammography, clinical breast examination, and colorectal cancer screening.

Of these studies, 10 are RCTs [15, 17-22, 61-63, 103, 104, 106-113] and 5 are observational studies [59, 60, 108, 113, 116, 125]. The RCTs include three randomized by communities [103] or churches [19-22, 104, 107]. Of the five observational studies, one was a quasi-experimental controlled cohort [125], two were prospective cohorts [108, 113], one used retrospective records [59, 60], and one used repeated cross- sectional survey of women attending beauty salons randomly assigned to experimental and control groups [116]. The studies spanned the quality range as well: two were of good quality [17, 18, 103], seven of fair quality [59-63, 106, 108, 109, 125], and six of poor quality [15, 19-22, 104, 107, 110-113, 116].

As noted in our section on KQ 1, seven studies used low-intensity CHW models, 6 used moderate-intensity interventions, and two used high-intensity interventions. Six studies included more than two arms. Studies compared the CHW arm with a variety of alternatives, including no intervention or usual care (6 studies), mail (3 studies), community interventions (4 studies), CHWs in a lesser capacity (2 studies), and CHWs in combination with other interventions (2 studies).

With the exception of two studies on colorectal cancer screening [106, 107], all other studies focus on women. All studies focused mainly on minority or underserved communities.

Studies used varied definitions of outcomes. The greatest commonality was reporting on utilization of cancer screening tests such as mammography, clinical breast examination, Pap smears, and colorectal cancer screening. Of the 15 studies, 13 reported on changes in rates of utilization, but they varied in their specific definitions (ever use, use in the past 3 months, 1 year, 2 years, and so on) [15, 17-22, 59-63, 104, 106-113, 125]. With the exception of 3 studies examining Medicaid or medical records for mammography use [17, 18, 59, 60, 63], all relied solely on self-report.

Overview of results. Together, the 15 studies suggest limited evidence of improvement in knowledge in the CHW arm compared with alternative approaches; they present conflicting findings on the effect of CHWs on planned and actual health behaviors, specifically breast self- examination. The volume of evidence on these outcomes is limited; the quality and design of the studies limits the interpretation of available evidence.

Unlike most of the other subsections dealing with other purposes for CHW strategies, cancer screening studies used high-, moderate-, and low-intensity interventions. Enough studies and evidence are available to permit some analysis by the intensity variable as it relates to Pap smears and mammography. Summary tables for these two outcomes are therefore presented by intensity (low, then moderate, then high), followed by quality, and then alphabetical order, by last name of first author(s); for all other sections, we present studies by quality, and then alphabetical order, by last name of first author(s).

Regarding health care utilization, our findings from this limited evidence do not support the conclusion that CHW interventions are more effective in comparison with other alternatives in raising the rates of clinical breast examination or colorectal cancer screening. More substantial evidence exists on Pap smears and mammography. The CHW approach is at least as effective as the alternative in improving Pap smear rates, but it is more effective than the alternative only in limited circumstances of low- and moderate-intensity interventions. With respect to mammography rates, studies demonstrated significantly greater improvements in the CHW arm compared with the alternative (no intervention, mail, print, or minimal CHW) in either the entire sample or in subsamples.

Table 18. CHW cancer screening: improving knowledge

Author, Year Study Design Population Setting Sample Size Quality	Intensity of CHW Intervention	Study Groups	Results
Paskett et al., 2006; [17] Katz et al., 2007 [18] RCT Community health centers, Robeson County, North Carolina 820 Good	High	G1: Letter and NCI brochure sent about the need for regular cervical cancer screening 6 months after random assignment, followed by letter and NCI brochure about the need for mammography 3 months after followup assessment (control) G2: Individualized health education program that was culturally acceptable and tailored to meet the needs of each woman, intensive face-to-face interactive educational program administered over a 9- to 12-month period, consisting of 3 in-person visits, with educational materials provided at each visit and followup telephone calls and mailings thereafter	Composite knowledge score: not statistically significantly higher in CHW group
Mock et al., 2007 [109] RCT Vietnamese-American women, Santa Clara County, California 968 Fair	Moderate	G1: CHW small group meetings; direct contact with subjects; Vietnamese language ads for TV, radio, newspaper; booklets and printed materials in various community locations G2: Vietnamese-language ads for TV, radio, newspaper; booklets and printed materials in various community locations; delayed educational session	Reported awareness of need for Pap test by women 18+ years old (baseline/followup): G1: 68.4%/93.9% ($P <$ 0.001) G2: 68.5%/70.2% ($P =$ 0.55) Z-test $P < 0.001$ Heard of Pap test: G1: 81.8%/99.6% ($P < 0.001$) G2: 87.2%/95.2% ($P <$ 0.001) Z-test $P < 0.001$

CHW, community health workers; G, group; NCI, National Cancer Institute; RCT, randomized controlled trial; TV, television.

Table 19. CHW cancer screening: changing planned behaviors

Author, Year Study Design Population Setting Sample Size Quality	Intensity of CHW Intervention	Study Groups	Results
Taylor, et al., 2002 [63] RCT Chinese-American women, Seattle, Washington, and Vancouver, British Columbia 402 (181 Seattle, 221 Vancouver) Fair	Low	G1: Introductory mailing, CHW visit with multimedia and tailored counseling, telephone followup and tailored counseling, logistic assistance as needed G2: Direct mail multimedia materials G3: Usual care at local clinics and doctors' offices (control)	Pap testing planned within 2 years: G1: 72% G2: 59% G3: 48% (G1 vs. G3 $P < 0.001$, G2 vs. G3 $P = 0.05$, G1 vs. G2 $P= 0.03$)
Wilson et al., 2008 [116] Repeated cross-sectional survey of women attending salons randomly assigned to experimental and control groups Neighborhood hair salons, Brooklyn, New York 40 salons/1,210 respondents Poor	Moderate	G1: Control, before intervention G2: Stylist group, before intervention G3: Control, after intervention G4: Stylist group, after intervention Intervention consisted of education, counseling, and information on location of screening services during salon appointment	Intention to receive clinical breast examination in next year:G3: 90% G4: 89% AOR, 0.9; adjusted 95% CI, 0.6-1.2 Intention to receive mammogramin next year: G3: 70% G4: 74% AOR, 1.3; adjusted 95% CI, 0.9-1.2

CHW, community health worker; CI, confidence interval; G, group; AOR, adjusted odds ratio.

Knowledge. Two studies (three articles; Table 18) examined changes in knowledge and found limited evidence of improvement for the CHW arm [17, 18, 109]. A good-quality, high-intensity study in North Carolina measured knowledge for 12 individual measures on breast cancer and a composite score [17, 18]. The studies together suggest improvements in the CHW arm, although the results are not consistent on the relative benefit of the CHW arm versus the alternative. Although differences between the CHW and the comparison arm (mail intervention) were not statistically significant for the composite measure of knowledge, the study reported significant different improvements favoring the CHW arm on two individual items measuring knowledge. Both arms demonstrated improvements in other measures, but these improvements were not statistically significantly different. A second study, of fair quality and moderate intensity in California, found significantly different improvements on two measures of knowledge, favoring the CHW arm compared with the media intervention arm [109].

Behavior: planned testing. Two studies, one of fair quality and low intensity [63] and the other of poor quality and moderate intensity [116], provide contradictory findings on the effect of CHWs on planned behavior Table 19). The fair-quality study compared a CHW arm with direct and usual care; differences in the rate of planned Pap smear tests favoring the CHW arm were statistically significant compared with either direct mail or usual care [63]. The poor-quality study reported no differences among study arms. However, the design of the study, which involved repeated cross-sections in salons randomly assigned to experimental and control status in which experimental salons offered barrier-specific counseling, was not measuring changes in intent over time; rather, it was concerned with differences in a cross-sectional sample. Low penetration combined with contamination across the samples (as suggested by the 37 percent and 10 percent of the sample reporting breast health messages at control sites and experimental sites, respectively) could have diluted the effects of the intervention [116].

Behavior: breast self-examination. Five studies (eight citations; Table 20) reported on changes in self-breast examination as outcomes of CHW interventions [61, 62, 108, 110-112, 116, 125]. Of these five studies, three were of fair quality [61, 62, 108, 125] and two of poor quality [110-112, 116]. They included one high-intensity [61, 62], three moderate-intensity [110-112, 116, 125], and one low-intensity study [108].

These studies provide conflicting evidence of the effectiveness of the CHW approach, either in comparison with an alternative or over time independent of a comparison. Two studies reported significant differences between the CHW arm and an alternative (low-intensity CHW, mailed intervention, delayed intervention, or no intervention) [108, 110-112]. The same two studies also provided evidence of significant differences between baseline and followup for the CHW arm [108, 110-112]. A third study employed repeated cross-sectional measurements and reported higher rates in the followup assessment but these were not statistically significant [116]. The fourth study failed to find any improvements over time [61, 62]. The fifth study found reported conflicting results for the two selected measures.

Of the three fair-quality studies, the high-intensity study compared the CHW arm with a mailed intervention [61, 62], the moderate-intensity study compared the CHW arm (outreach) to no- intervention arm, and the low-intensity CHW arm compared the CHW arm to a delayed intervention [108]. The high-intensity study found no significant improvements over time in either arm, or between arms, except when the sample was restricted to a much reduced subsample who were available at followup and were not on the recommended screening schedule [61, 62]. The moderate-intensity study found improvements in the intervention arm over time for ever use of breast self-examination, but no significant differences in the control arm, but also found opposite effects for another measure: monthly breast self-examinations, with significant differences in the control arm over time, but not the intervention arm The low-intensity study found that the CHW arm resulted in significant improvements over time compared with the delayed-intervention arm [108]. However, baseline differences between the two arms were large; significant differences between the two arms could have resulted from ceiling effects.

Of the two poor-quality studies, one moderate-intensity intervention compared a more intense CHW arm with a less intense CHW arm; [110-112] the other moderate-intensity intervention compared the CHW arm with a no-intervention control [116]. In the former study, the two arms differed significantly through 1-year followup but not at the 2-year followup [110-112]. In the latter study, rates of breast self-examination were higher in followup interviews than in baseline interviews, but the differences between the arms was not statistically significant [116].

Table 20. CHW cancer screening: changing breast self-examination behavior

Author, Year Study Design Population Setting Sample Size Quality	Intensity of CHW Intervention	Study Groups	Results
Erwin et al., 1997 [108] Prospective cohort Church or community groups, rural Mississippi River Delta region, Arkansas 412 Fair	Low	G1: Members of a Witness Project team, composed of 7 local African-American women who had survived breast or cervical cancer, spoke in groups of 2 to 5 at local churches and community organization meetings G2: Delayed intervention (control)	Regular practice of BSE (self-report): G1: 69.8% to 82% ($P <$ 0.005 compared with baseline) G2: 82% to 82% (P = NS compared with baseline) BSE in the past month (self-report): G1: 49% to 65.4% ($P < 0.001$ compared with baseline) G2: 65% to 72% (P = NS compared with baseline)
Hiatt et al., 2008 [125] Prospective cohort Public health clinics and the low-income neighborhoods in San Francisco and Contra Costa County, California 1,616 Fair	Moderate	G1: One-on-one visits at various events and locations; presentations to community-based organizations (agencies); and Women's Health Days, offering free mammograms, Pap tests, and breast self-examination instruction G2: No intervention (control)	Ever completed breast self-examination (Total N [%] pretest/Total N [%] posttest): G1: 800 (89)/810 (92) X2 = NR, $P = 0.031$ G2: 793 (83)/ 802(81) X^2 = NR, not significant Completed breast self-examination monthly in the past year (Total N [%] pretest/Total N [%] posttest): G1: 800 (24)/808 (26) X^2 = NR, not significant G2: 793 (18)/ 801(23) X^2 = NR, $P = 0.018$
Sung et al., 1997 [61]; Sung et al., 1992 [62] RCT Inner-city African Americans, state unspecified 195 Fair	High	G1: CHW home visits, education on breast and cervical cancer, BSE educational materials on screening, facilitation to address logistical barriers to screening G2: Mailed educational materials on cancer screening	Pretest/posttest change in self-report of BSE for entire sample: G1: 52.1%/51.0% G2: 41.1%/41.0%, difference in change: -1.0 (95% CI, -6.1 to 4.1) Pretest/posttest change in self-report of BSE, postintervention respondents only:G1: 57.0%/53.8% G2: 40.2%/40.2%, difference in change: -3.2 (95% CI, -17.5 to 11.1) Posttest report of BSE, women not previously on recommended screening schedules, whole sample: G1: 24.4% G2: 17.2%, difference in change: 7.2% (95% CI, -5.0-19.3) Posttest report of BSE, women not previously on recommended screening schedules, postintervention respondents only: G1: 47.5% G2: 26.2%, difference in change: 21.3% (95% CI, 2.3-40.3)
Navarro et al., 1998, [111] Navarro et al., 1995, [110] Navarro et al., 2000 [112] RCT Low-income Latinas,	Moderate	G1: CHW delivering community living skills sessions, details NR G2: CHW delivering cancer education sessions, 12 weekly group sessions conducted over 3 months	Pretest-posttest changes in percentage of women performing monthly BSEs: Participant unit of analysis (n = 361) G1: 18.5 G2: 33.2 $P < 0.001$

Table 20. (Continued)

Author, Year Study Design Population Setting Sample Size Quality	Intensity of CHW Intervention	Study Groups	Results
Southeast San Diego County, California 365 Poor		plus 2 additional sessions offered within a year of beginning of group meetings	t = 3.23 CHW unit of analysis (n = 35) G1: 18.6 G2: 31.8 *P* = 0.021 t = 2.43 Odds of monthly BSE at 1-year and 2-year followup for cancer screening group (*P* value): Year 1: 2.03 (0.016) Year 2: 0.96 (0.877)
Wilson et al., 2008 [116] Repeated cross-sectional survey of women attending salons randomly assigned to experimental and control groups Neighborhood hair salons, Brooklyn, New York 40 salons/1,210 respondents Poor	Moderate	G1: Control, before intervention G2: Stylist group, before intervention G3: Control, after intervention G4: Stylist group, after intervention Intervention: provide messages promoting breast health during salon visit	Engaging in BSE in past 3 months: G1: 25% G2: 28%, *P* = 0.26 for differences between G1 and G2 G3: 37% G4: 40% AOR for differences between G3 and G41.3; adjusted 95% CI, 0.9-1.7

AOR, adjusted odds ratio; BSE, breast self examination; CHW, community health worker; CI, confidence interval; G, group; NR, not reported; NS, not significant; OR, odds ratio; RCT, randomized controlled trial.

Satisfaction. No study reported outcomes for satisfaction.

Health outcomes: No study reported on health outcomes.

Health care utilization: Pap smears. The evidence on the effectiveness of CHW interventions draws upon six studies (nine articles; Table 21) [17, 18, 61-63, 110-112]. Most studies demonstrate that the CHW arm is as effective as the alternative in improving Pap smear rates. CHWs were not more effective than mailed interventions in high-intensity interventions. They were more effective than the alternative in limited circumstances involving low- or moderate- intensity intervention in three of four studies. Because intensity may, thus, actually be an important policy variable for analyzing use of Pap smears, we present information on Pap smear use ordered first by intensity and then by the quality of the studies.

One low-intensity trial, of fair quality, compared CHWs with direct mail and with usual care in cities in Washington and British Columbia [63]. CHWs were more effective than either alternative in increasing Pap smear rates, using both self-report and medical records.

Of the three moderate-intensity interventions, one in Santa Clara County, California, was of fair quality [109], a second in San Francisco and Contra Costa was also fair quality [125], and the third in San Diego County, California, was rated poor quality [110-112]. The fair-quality study in Santa Clara compared CHWs with a media intervention; CHWs were effective in increasing rates of Pap smears [109]. The fair-quality study in San Francisco and

Contra Costa found no statistically significant difference in changes in self-reported Pap smears between residents of intervention and control communities [125]. The poor-quality study compared a higher-intensity CHW arm focusing on cancer control with a lower-intensity CHW arm [110-112]. Although both arms demonstrated effectiveness compared with baseline values, participation in the more intense arm did not affect use of Pap smears compared with the less intense arm in the short term, but it did demonstrate effectiveness in the longer term (at 1- and 2-year followups). Followups were marked by high dropout rates, however, so the effectiveness in the longer term could be explained by selection bias.

Table 21. CHW cancer screening: Pap smears

Author, Year Study Design Population Setting Sample Size Quality	Intensity of CHW Intervention	Study Groups	Results
Taylor, et al., 2002 [63] RCT Chinese-American women, Seattle, Washington, and Vancouver, British Columbia 402 (181 Seattle, 221 Vancouver) Fair	Low	G1: Introductory mailing, CHW visit with multimedia and tailored counseling, telephone followup and tailored counseling, logistic assistance as needed G2: Direct mail multimedia materials G3: Usual care at local clinics and doctors' offices (control)	Self-reported Pap testing completed since intervention: G1: 39%, G2: 25%, G3: 15% (G1 vs. G3, *P* < 0.001; G2 vs. G3, *P*= 0.03; G1 vs. G2, *P* = 0.02) Medical records for Pap screening received between randomization and followup, using intention-to-treat: Results not provided, significant differences between outreach worker versus control (*P* <.001), direct mail versus control (*P* =.07), and outreach worker versus direct mail (*P* =.04) Medical records for Pap screening received in the past 2 years, using intention-to-treat: Results not provided, significant differences between outreach worker versus control (*P* <.001) and direct mailversus control (*P* =.03)
Hiatt et al., 2008 [125] Prospective cohort Public health clinics and the low-income neighborhoods in San Francisco and Contra Costa County, California 1,616 Fair	Moderate	G1: One-on-one visits at various events and locations; presentations to community-based organizations (agencies); and Women's Health Days, offering free mammograms, Pap tests, and breast self-examination instruction G2: No intervention (control)	Ever completed Pap smear (logistic regression, 95% CI) Residence in outreach area over time: 1.5(0.6-4.2) Completed Pap smear in the past 3 years (logistic regression, 95% CI) Residence in outreach area over time: 0.9(0.6-1.3)
Mock et al., 2007 [109] RCT Vietnamese-American women, Santa Clara County, California 968 Fair	Moderate	G1: CHW small group meetings, direct contact with subjects, Vietnamese language ads for TV/radio/newspaper, booklets and printed materials in various community locations G2: Vietnamese-language ads for TV/radio/newspaper, booklets and printed materials in various community locations, delayed educational session	Self-report of having ever had Pap (baseline/followup): G1: 65.8%/81.8% (*P* < 0.001); G2: 70.1%/75.5% (*P* < 0.001); Z test P = 0.001 Self-report of Pap in past year: G1: 45.7%/67.3% (*P* < 0.001); G2: 50.9%/55.7% (*P* = 0.035); Z test *P* < 0.001 Ever had Pap test (among those who had not had Pap test pre-outreach): G1: 46.0 (N = 144); G2: 27.1 (N = 161) *P* < 0.001

Table 21. (Continued)

Author, Year Study Design Population Setting Sample Size Quality	Intensity of CHW Intervention	Study Groups	Results
Navarro et al., 1998; [111] Navarro et al., 1995; [110] Navarro et al., 2000 [112] RCT Low-income Latinas, southeast San Diego County, California 365 Poor	Moderate	G1: CHW delivering community living skills sessions, details NR G2: CHW delivering cancer education sessions, 12 weekly group sessions conducted over 3 months plus 2 additional sessions offered within a year of beginning of group meetings	Pretest-posttest changes in percentages of women who had a Paptest within past year: Participant unit of analysis (n = 360) G1: 16.2 G2: 23.1 $P = 0.096$ t = 1.67 CHW unit of analysis (n = 35) G1: 18.4 G2: 23.4 $P = 0.369$ t = 0.91 Odds of Pap smear 1-year and 2-year followup for cancer screening group (*P* value): Year 1: 2.10 (0.017) Year 2: 1.70 (0.082)
Paskett et al., 2006; [17] Katz et al., 2007 [18] RCT Community health centers, Robeson County, North Carolina 820 Good	High	G1: Control sent letter and NCI brochure about the need for regular cervical cancer screening 6 months after random assignment, followed by letter and NCI brochure about the need for mammography 3 months after followup assessment G2: Individualized health education program that was culturally acceptable and tailored to meet the needs of each woman, intensive face-to-face interactive educational program administered over a 9- to 12-month period, consisting of 3 in-person visits, with educational materials provided each visit and followup telephone calls and mailings after	Cervical cancer screening rates within risk-appropriate guidelines: Significant differences between baseline and followup for both groups, no significant differences between intervention and control groups
Sung et al., 1997; [61] Sung et al., 1992 [62] RCT Inner-city African Americans, state unspecified 195 Fair	High	G1: CHW home visits, education on breast and cervical cancer, breast self-exam, educational materials on screening, facilitation to address logistical barriers to screening G2: Mailed educational materials on cancer screening	Pretest/posttest change in self-report of receiving Pap smears for entire sample: G1: 50.3%/58.7% G2: 51.9%/62.1%, difference in change: -1.8 (95% CI, -8.0-4.4) Pretest/posttest change in self-report of receiving Pap smears, postintervention respondents only: G1: 52.7%/63.4% G2: 50.0%/62.7%, difference in change: -2.0 (95% CI, -11.0-7.0) Posttest rate of self-report of receiving Pap smears, women not previously on

Author, Year Study Design Population Setting Sample Size Quality	Intensity of CHW Intervention	Study Groups	Results
			recommended screening schedules, whole sample: G1: 33.3% G2: 34.2%, difference in change: -0.9 (95% CI, -15.7-13.9) Posttest rate of self-report of receiving Pap smears, women not previously on recommended screening schedules, postintervention respondents only: G1: 61.4% G2: 51.0%, difference in change: 10.4 (95% CI, -9.5-30.0)

CHW, community health worker; CI, confidence interval; G, group; N, number; NCI, National Cancer Institute; NR, not reported; RCT, randomized controlled trial; TV, television.

Two high-intensity trials, one good-quality study in North Carolina [17, 18], and one fair-quality study among inner-city African Americans (location unspecified) [61, 62], compared CHWs to mailed interventions. These two studies reported consistent results failing to demonstrate effectiveness of CHWs in improving Pap smear use compared with mailed interventions, but both studies showed that both arms demonstrated improvement compared with baseline values.

Health care utilization: mammography. Eleven studies (21 articles; Table 22), provide evidence on the effectiveness of CHW intervention with respect to breast cancer screening by mammography [15, 17-22, 59-62, 103, 104, 108, 110-113, 116]. Eight of these studies demonstrated significantly greater improvements in the CHW arm compared with the alternative (no intervention, mail, print, or minimal CHW) in either the entire sample or in subsamples [17-22, 59-62, 103, 104, 108, 110-113]. Two of three studies reporting nonsignificant differences between the CHW arm and the alternative were moderate-intensity, poor-quality studies comparing CHWs with no intervention; [15, 116] one of these studies reported nonsignificant differences between the CHW arm and the control, favoring the CHW arm. The third was a moderate-intensity fair-quality study comparing the effect of CHW interventions with controls at the community level [125]. As with use of Pap smears, intensity may be a relevant analytic variable, so we report findings below first by intensity, then by study quality.

Four studies did not report changes over time; [15, 17-22, 103, 104] one study failed to show improvement in the intervention area [125], and the remaining six studies all demonstrated some improvement in the control arm (no intervention, delayed intervention, mail, print, or minimal CHW), although the improvement was not statistically significant.

Studies conducting subgroup analyses demonstrated that CHW interventions can provide benefits for subpopulations. Four studies provide evidence that CHW interventions are likely to be more beneficial than alternative interventions in low-income, minority populations with some health care barriers [19-22, 60, 103, 104, 113].

Low-intensity interventions generally compared CHW with minimal to no intervention, We identified five such studies, one good-quality [103], two fair [59, 60, 108], and two poor [19-22, 104, 113]. Collectively CHWs were generally effective in raising mammography rates, but with potentially greater effects in subpopulations.

The good study from Washington State, comparing a no-intervention control group with CHW groups receiving community activities, individual counseling, or a combination of community activities and individual counseling found that all the CHW intervention arms had higher rates of new users than the no-intervention control, but the study did not find significantly greater effectiveness of CHW arms in comparison with a no-intervention control [103] The community activities arm appeared to be more effective than a no-intervention control in preventing relapse (that is, in ensuring that regular users or women who were adherent to recommended screening guidelines at baseline continued to be adherent at followup) than in enrolling new users.

One fair-quality study involved Latinas in Colorado enrolled in Medicare or Medicaid fee- for-service, or three other health maintenance organizations (Kaiser Permanente of Colorado, Access, and Anthem Blue Cross and Blue Shield) [59]. It found nonsignificant and modest differences in mammography screening rates in unadjusted analyses that compared a CHW intervention with a printed intervention. In adjusted analysis, the difference between the two arms was statistically significant, favoring the CHW arm. The other fair-quality study, in Arkansas, also reported significantly greater improvements in self-reported use of mammography in the CHW arm compared with a delayed intervention arm. However, the two groups differed significantly at baseline, with higher rates of ever-use of mammography reported in the control group; thus a ceiling effect limiting improvements in the control group cannot be ruled out [108].

The two poor-quality, low-intensity studies also suggested favorable results for the CHW arm compared with a minimal [19-22, 104] or no-intervention arm [113] for the entire sample or for subpopulations.

Four moderate-intensity interventions, one of fair quality [125] and three of poor quality [15, 110-112, 116], reported outcomes for self-reported mammography use. The fair-quality study in San Francisco and Contra Costa found no statistically significant difference in changes in self- reported mammography between intervention communities and control communities [125]. One study in New York, which compared CHW with no-intervention controls, found no significant differences between intervention and control arms after the intervention in use of mammography during the prior 3 months [116]. Both studies described measure effects at the community level rather than at the individual level. Low penetration of the intervention and potential contamination between experimental and control samples limit the interpretation of the results.

Two other studies, both assessed as moderate intensity overall, compared higher-intensity CHW to lower-intensity CHW intervention; [15, 110-112] they both reported improvements in both arms. Only the study in San Diego County, California, found significant differences; it demonstrated that the relatively more intense arm was more effective in the 3- to 6-month period following the intervention [110-112]. These improvements were not consistently significantly different between the two arms over the long run (1- and 2-year followups) for a reduced and potentially self-selected subsample.

Table 22. CHW cancer screening: mammography

Author, Year Study Design Population Setting Sample Size Quality	Intensity of CHW Intervention	Study Groups	Results
Andersen, 2000 [103] RCT of communities Rural communities, Washington 6,685 Good	Low	G1: Control—no intervention reported G2: Community activities—developing social norms G3: Individual counseling—telephone G4: Community activities and individual counseling	Proportion of mammography rates among regular users (regular user is more than 1 mammogram, last mammogram within 2 years, and the previous mammogram within 2 years of the last mammogram) (self-reported): G1: 0.922 G2: 0.951, difference from G1 = 0.029, $P = 0.01$ (95% CI, 0.008-0.052) G3: 0.918, difference from G1 = 0.004, $P = 0.81$ (95% CI, -0.043-0.032) G4: 0.936, difference from G1 = 0.014, $P = 0.27$ (95% CI, -0.013-0.039) Proportion for G2+G3+G4: 0.935, difference from G1 = 0.013, $P = 0.40$ (95% CI, -0.012-0.038) In subgroup analysis, the intervention was more effective than the control in preventing relapse among women who needed >2 hours to get a medical appointment G1: 88.1%, difference in proportions for G2: 7.1% ($P \leq 0.01$) G2: 6.0% ($P \leq 0.01$) G3: 5.6% ($P \leq 0.05$) Proportion of mammography rates among new users (under-users at baseline) (self-reported): G1: 0.578 G2: 0.599, difference from G1 = 0.021, $P = 0.63$ (95% CI, -0.080-0.117) G3: 0.606, difference from G1 = 0.028, $P = 0.47$ (95% CI, -0.064-0.113) G4: 0.604, difference from G1 = 0.026,

Table 22. (Continued)

Author, Year Study Design Population Setting Sample Size Quality	Intensity of CHW Intervention	Study Groups	Results
			$P = 0.55$ (95% CI, -0.062-0.122) Proportion for G2+G3+G4: 0.603, difference from G1 = 0.025, $P = 0.40$ (95% CI, -0.035-0.085) In subgroup analysis, among under-users/intervention more effective than control in increasing mammography rates among women within communities without a female physician (G2: 12.4%, G3: 10.5%, G4: 16.5%; $P < 0.05$) and among women with no health insurance (G2: 23.2%, G3: 9.9%, G4: 22.1%; $P \leq 0.05$)
Erwin et al., 1997 [108] Prospective cohort Church or community groups, rural Mississippi River Delta region, Arkansas 412 Fair	Low	G1: Members of a Witness Project team, composed of 7 local African-American women who had survived breast or cervical cancer, spoke in groups of 2 to 5 at local churches and community organization meetings G2: Delayed intervention (control)	Ever had mammography (self-report): G1: 52.4% to 64.4% ($P < 0.05$ compared with baseline) G2: 60.4% to 63.3% (P = NS compared with baseline)
Sauaia et al., 2007; [59] Welsh et al., 2005 [60] Retrospective cohort Church communities, Colorado Latina-only analysis: 4,739 [59]; Latina vs. white analysis: 6,696 [60] Fair	Low	G1: Trained peer counselors (Promotoras) delivered health promotion message personally, through meetings held at least bimonthly immediately after mass and through other church events, conducted health groups that met at the home of one of the participants, same newsletter used in the printed intervention G2: Printed intervention incorporated into church display, bulletin, and/or pulpit announcements	Pretest/posttest mammography rates via ICD codes on Medicaid claims (baseline/followup): Latina-only analysis: G1: 59%/61% G2: 58%/58%, unadjusted rates not significant in either group, GEE model adjusting for insurance group, age, income, rural vs. urban, and disability found increased biennial mammograms in intervention group ($P = 0.03$)[59] Latina vs. white analysis: G1: Latina 25%/30% (unadjusted GEE $P = 0.3$);

Author, Year Study Design Population Setting Sample Size Quality	Intensity of CHW Intervention	Study Groups	Results
			non-Latina 32%/38% (unadjusted GEE $P = 0.4$) G2: Latina 45%/43% (unadjusted GEE $P = 0.27$); non-Latina 41%/44% (unadjusted GEE $P = 0.02$)[60] Comparison of mammography rates by intervention and ethnicity, via ICD codes on Medicaid claims (pretest-posttest time-intervention interaction term by GEE) Latina: G1 vs. G2 adjusted GEE $P = 0.07$ Non-Latina: G1 vs. G2 adjusted GEE $P = 0.10$
Derose et al., 2000; [19] Dean et al., 2000; [20] Derose et al., 2000; [21] Stockdale et al., 2000; [22] Fox et al., 1998 [104] RCT Church communities, Louisiana 813 Poor	Low	G1: Control churches provided minimal intervention: a library of resource materials on cancer and cancer prevention; assistance with starting a health committee or working with an existing health committee; computer hardware, software, and a printer, as well as computer training for at least 1 church member G2: 1 session of telephone counseling annually, for 2 years, by peer counselor; counseling individualized to address barriers; churches also received computer support offered to control churches	Nonadherence rate (among baseline adherent): G1: 23.3% G2: 15.8% ($P = 0.029$) Nonadherence rate (among baseline nonadherent): G1: 37.4% G2: 34.8% ($P = 0.324$)
Earp et al., 2002 [113] Prospective cohort Black women, eastern North Carolina 801 Poor	Low	G1: Counties receiving CHW and other targeted activity—presentations to community groups and events, one-on-one conversations, use of informational/motivational materials G2: Comparison counties—no intervention reported	Self-report of mammogram in past 2 years (baseline/followup): G1: 41%/58% G2: 56%/67% (adjusted $P = 0.05$) Self-report of mammogram in past 2 years, stratified by income (baseline/ followup): < $12k annually— G1: 37%/59% G2: 49%/60% (adjusted $P = 0.02$) $12k or greater annually— G1: 56%/59% G2: 73%/82% (adjusted $P = 0.92$)

Table 22. (Continued)

Author, Year Study Design Population Setting Sample Size Quality	Intensity of CHW Intervention	Study Groups	Results
Dignan et al., 2005 [15] RCT Urban American-Indian women, Denver, Colorado 157 (for intervention groups, N for control NR) Poor	Moderate	G1: Control interventions NR data from Colorado Mammography Program G2: Tailored education brochure using data from baseline interview. Face-to-face planned for delivery at participant's home (1 session lasting 20-90 minutes), presenting information on breast cancer and value of early detection, review of brochure G3: Telephone intervention, as above	Mammograms over past 12 months, self-report (baseline/followup): G1: 51.9%/50.0% G2: 29%/41.8% G3: 34.4%/45.2% Chi-square: G1 vs. G2+G3: 2.68, P = 0.10; *P* for G2 vs. G3: 0.83; *P* for G2, pre-changes: 0.029; *P* for G3, pre-changes: 0.197
Hiatt et al., 2008 [125] Prospective cohort Public health clinics and the low-income neighborhoods in San Francisco and Contra Costa County, California 1,616 Fair	Moderate	G1: One-on-one visits at various events and locations; presentations to community-based organizations (agencies); and Women's Health Days, offering free mammograms, Pap tests, and breast self-examination instruction G2: No intervention (control)	Ever completed mammography (logistic regression, 95% CI) Residence in outreach area over time: 0.7 (0.5-1.0) Completed mammography in past 2 years (logistic regression, 95% CI) Residence in outreach area over time: 0.7 (0.5-1.0) Completed 3 mammographies in past 5 years (logistic regression, 95% CI) Residence in outreach area over time: 0.8 (0.5-1.1)
Navarro et al., 1998; [111]	Moderate	G1: CHW delivering community living skills sessions, details NR	Pretest-posttest changes in percentage of women 40 years who had mammogram within past year:
Navarro et al., 1995; [110] Navarro et al., 2000 [112] RCT Low-income Latinas, southeast San Diego County, California 365 Poor		G2: CHW delivering cancer education sessions, 12 weekly group sessions conducted over 3 months plus 2 additional sessions offered within a year of beginning of group meetings	Participant unit of analysis (n = 113) G1: 7 G2: 21.4 P = 0.029 t = 2.22 CHW unit of analysis (n = 33) G1: 6.8 G2: 24.3 P = 0.063 t = 1.96 Odds of mammogram 1-year and 2-year

Author, Year Study Design Population Setting Sample Size Quality	Intensity of CHW Intervention	Study Groups	Results
			followup for cancer screening group (*P* value):Year 1: 1.50 (0.484) Year 2: 3.88 (0.018)
Wilson et al., 2008 [116] Repeated cross-sectional survey of women attending salons randomly assigned to experimental and control groups Neighborhood hair salons, Brooklyn, New York 40 salons/1,210 Respondents Poor	Moderate	Intervention consisted of education, counseling, and information on location of screening services during salon appointment G1: Control, before intervention G2: Stylist group, before intervention G3: Control, after intervention G4: Stylist group, after intervention	Mammogram in past 3 months: G1: 13% G2: 14% AOR, 1.1 (95% CI, 0.8-1.7)
Paskett et al., 2006; [17] Katz et al., 2007 [18] RCT Community health centers, Robeson County,	High	G1: Sent control letter and NCI brochure about the need for regular cervical cancer screening 6 months after random assignment, followed by letter and NCI brochure about the need for mammography 3 months after followup assessment G2: Individualized health education program that was culturally acceptable and tailored to meet the needs of	Mammogram receipt from medical record data: G1: 27.3% G2: 42.5%, RR, 1.56; 95% CI, 1.29-1.87, $P<.001$
North Carolina 820 Good		each woman, intensive face-to-face interactive educational program administered over a 9- to 12-month period, consisting of 3 in-person visits, with educational materials provided each visit and followup telephone calls and mailings after	Significant differences within racial groups as well
Sung et al., 1997; [61] Sung et al., 1992 [62] RCT Inner-city African Americans, state unspecified 195 Fair	High	G1: CHW home visits, education on breast and cervical cancer, breast self-exam, educational materials on screening, facilitation to address logistical barriers to screening G2: Mailed educational materials on cancer screening	Pretest/posttest change in self- report of receiving mammography for entire sample: G1: 35.5%/50.4% G2: 34.3%/39.4%, difference in change: 9.8% (95% CI, 2.9-16.7) Pretest/posttest change in self- report of receiving mammography, post intervention respondents only: G1: 32.5%/58.7% G2: 34.0%/47.9%, difference in

Table 22. (Continued)

Author, Year Study Design Population Setting Sample Size Quality	Intensity of CHW Intervention	Study Groups	Results
			change: 12.4% (95% CI, 1.0-24.3) Posttest rate of self-report of receiving mammography, women not previously on recommended screening schedules, whole sample: G1: 29.7% G2: 24.4%, difference in change: 5.8% (95% CI, -7.0-18.6) Posttest rate of self-report of receiving mammography, women not previously on recommended screening schedules, post intervention respondents only: G1: 50.0% G2: 35.5%, difference in change: 14.5% (95% CI, 4.5-23.6)

CHW, community health worker; CI, confidence interval; G, group; GEE, generalized estimating equation; ICD, International Classification of Diseases; N, number; NCI, National Cancer Institute; NR, not reported; NS, not significant; OR, odds ratio; RCT, randomized controlled trial; RR, relative risk; t, t-test.

Two high-intensity trials, one good-quality [17, 18] and one fair-quality [61, 62], both compared CHWs to mailed interventions and reported improvements in the CHW arms of their studies. Only the good-quality study (using Medicaid records from North Carolina) found significant differences in mammography rates between the CHW arm and the mailed intervention arm [17, 18]. The fair-quality study, using self-reported mammography among inner-city African Americans (location unspecified), did not find any significant differences for the overall sample using intention-to-treat analysis, but it did report significant differences when analysis was limited to a potentially biased subsample of respondents available at followup [62, 129].

Four studies found evidence of effect modification in subgroup analysis [19-22, 60, 103, 104, 113]. The evidence is derived from low-intensity studies of varying quality. The good-quality study from Washington found that CHW intervention arms were more effective than a control arm in subgroups: among regular users (women adherent at baseline), the CHW intervention arms showed significantly greater rates of mammography use among women who needed less than 2 hours to schedule a medical appointment [103]. In the same study, subgroup analysis for under-users (women who were not adherent at baseline) found that the CHW interventions were significantly more effective than the no-intervention control among women without female doctors or insurance. These subgroup findings suggest that the CHW approach is effective in addressing some, but not all, access barriers to the use of mammography.

The fair-quality study from Colorado [59, 60] reported weak but slightly more powerful effects of the CHW approach compared with a printed intervention approach in increasing mammography rates among Medicaid-enrolled Latinas compared with non-Latina whites (P = 0.07 for Latinas, and P = 0.10 for non-Latina whites) [60]. Similarly, the poor-quality studies also suggested subgroup effects. One study found CHWs to be more effective than a no-intervention control group in increasing rates of self-reported mammography for the overall sample and in groups with incomes below $12,000, but not in groups with incomes equal to or exceeding $12,000 [113]. Another found that the CHW approach was more effective than with a minimal intervention approach in ensuring conversion to adherence among under-users rather than in maintaining adherence among regular or adherent users [19-22, 104].

Health care utilization: clinical breast examination. Four studies reporting on clinical breast examination (seven articles; Table 23) [61, 62, 110-112, 116] included a high-intensity and three moderate- intensity interventions. Two of these studies were of fair quality; [61, 62, 125] the other two were rated poor [110-112, 116]. Together the studies suggest that CHW interventions are not effective in comparison with other alternatives, although two studies that provide information on changes between baseline and followup found that the CHW arm results in improvements over time.

The fair-quality high-intensity trial found no differences between the CHW arm and a mailed intervention, with the exception of a reduced and possibly selective sample of respondents only at followup [61, 62]. The fair-quality moderate-intensity study found no difference over time in most measures of self-reported clinical breast examination in intervention communities or control communities [125]. Of the two poor-quality moderate-intensity studies, one trial compared a more intense CHW arm with a less intense CHW arm [110-112] and the cross-sectional study compared it with a no-intervention arm [116]. Neither study reported significant differences, although the women in the more intense CHW arm of the trial did report higher rates of clinical breast examination after the intervention.

Health care utilization: colorectal cancer screening. Two studies, one of moderate intensity and fair quality, and another of low intensity and poor quality compared three groups on outcomes for fecal occult blood tests (FOBT) and other colorectal cancer screening tests (Table 24) [107]. In the fair-quality moderate-intensity intervention, patients who received navigation services had higher rates of FOBT after three months of services than patients who received usual care, but these differences were not statistically significant. Patients receiving navigation services were significantly more likely than controls to have set an endoscopy appointment at three months and kept it by six months after the intervention [106]. The low-intensity poor-quality study reported that rates of FOBT were higher in the CHW arm over time; however, the CHW arm and the comparison arms of a no-intervention control or of tailored print and videotapes did not differ significantly. The study reported no benefit of the intervention for other colorectal screening tests.

Table 23. CHW cancer screening: clinical breast examination

Author, Year Study Design Population Setting Sample Size Quality	Intensity of CHW Intervention	Study Groups	Results
Sung et al., 1997 [61]; Sung et al., 1992 [62] RCT Inner-city African Americans, state unspecified 195 Fair	High	G1: CHW home visits, education on breast and cervical cancer, breast self-exam, educational materials on screening, facilitation to address logistical barriers to screening G2: Mailed educational materials on cancer screening	Pretest/posttest change in self-report of receiving CBE for entire sample: G1: 55.2%/64.5% G2: 55.7%/59.5%, difference in change: 4.9 (95% CI, -6.1-4.1) Pretest/posttest change in self-report of receiving CBE, postintervention respondents only: G1: 59.1%/72.0% G2: 57.8%/61.8%, difference in change: 8.9% (95% CI, 1.1-16.7) Posttest rate of self-report of receiving CBE, women not previously on recommended screening schedules, whole sample: G1: 37.0% G2: 28.6%, difference in change: 8.4% (95% CI, -6.9-23.7) Posttest rate of self-report of receiving CBE, women not previously on recommended screening schedules, postintervention respondents only: G1: 71.1% G2: 46.5%, difference in change: 24.6% (95% CI, 3.9-45.3)
Hiatt et al., 2008 [125] Prospective Cohort Public health clinics and the low-income neighborhoods in San Francisco and Contra Costa County, California	Moderate	G1: One-on-one visits at various events and locations; presentations to community-based organizations (agencies); and Women's Health Days, offering free mammograms, Pap tests, and breast self-examination instruction	Ever completed clinical breast examination (Total N [%] pretest/Total N [%] posttest): G1: 801 (94)/812 (95) X^2 = NR, not significant G2: 798 (82)/ 803 (87) X^2 = NR, P = 0.006 Completed clinical breast examination in past year (Total N [%] pretest/Total N [%] posttest):

Author, Year Study Design Population Setting Sample Size Quality	Intensity of CHW Intervention	Study Groups	Results
1,616 Fair		G2: No intervention (control)	G1: 800 (75)/809 (74) X^2 = NR, not significant G2: 796 (56)/ 803 (60) X^2 = NR, not significant Completed 3 or more clinical breast examinations in past 5 years (Total N [%] pretest/Total N [%] posttest): G1: 793 (73)/809 (73) X^2 = NR, not significant G2: 792 (54)/ 800 (54) X^2 = NR, not significant
Navarro et al., 1998; [111] Navarro et al., 1995; [110] Navarro et al., 2000 [112] RCT Low-income Latinas, southeast San Diego County, California 365 Poor	Moderate	G1: CHW delivering community living skills sessions, details NR G2: CHW delivering cancer education sessions, 12 weekly group sessions conducted over 3 months plus 2 additional sessions offered within a year of beginning of group meetings	Pretest-posttest changes in percentage of women who had CBE within past year: Participant unit of analysis (n = 359) G1: 15.5 G2: 17.7 P = 0.589 t = 0.54 CHW unit of analysis (n = 35) G1: 19.3 G2: 19.5 P = 0.967 t = 0.04 Odds of CBE 1-year and 2-year followup for cancer screening group (P value): Year 1: 1.21 (0.556) Year 2: 1.93 (0.038)
Wilson et al., 2008 [116] Repeated cross-sectional survey of women attending salons randomly assigned to experimental and control groups Neighborhood hair salons, Brooklyn, New York 40 salons/1,210 respondents Poor	Moderate	Intervention consisted of education, counseling, and information on location of screening services during salon appointment G1: Control, before intervention G2: Stylist group, before intervention G3: Control, after intervention G4: Stylist group, after intervention	CBE in past 3 months: G1: 27% G2: 27%, P = 0.85 for differences between G1 and G2 G3: 27% G4: 29% AOR, 1.2; adjusted 95% CI, 0.9-1.7

Adj, adjusted; CBE, clinical breast examination; CHW, community health worker; CI, confidence interval; NR, not reported; OR, odds ratio; RCT, randomized controlled trial; t, t-test.

Table 24. CHW cancer screening: Colorectal cancer screening

Author, Year Study Design Population Setting Sample Size Quality	Intensity of CHW Intervention	Study Groups	Results
Jandorf et al., 2005 RCT East Harlem, New York City 78 Fair	Moderate	G1: Patient navigator (education and assistance with screening and navigation process) G2: Usual care	Completed FOBT after 3 months (%): G1: 42.1 G2: 25.0 $P = 0.086$ Had endoscopy appointment at 3 months (%): G1: 18.4 G2: 0 $P = 0.005$ Completed endoscopy at 3 months (%): G1: 15.8 G2: 5.0 $P = 0.115$ Completed endoscopy at 6 months (%): G1: 23.7 G2: 5.0 $P = 0.019$
Campbell, 2004 [107] RCT African-American rural churches, North Carolina NR (12 churches; completers/dropouts of individual participants from each church NR) Poor	Low	G1: Control churches were offered health education sessions and speakers on topics of their choice not directly related to study objectives G2: Organized and conducted at least 3 church-wide activities on spreading information and enhancing support for healthy lifestyle and CRC screening (LHA) G3: 4 personalized computer-tailored newsletters and 4 targeted videotapes corresponding to the same behaviors mailed to participants' homes bimonthly for first 6 months after baseline data collection; 4th targeted videotape mailing was 9 months after baseline G4: LHA and targeted videotapes	FOBT test in past year (% baseline/% followup): G1: 30.4%/21.7% G2: 23.5%/33.3% G3: 19.7%/36.8% G4: 19.5%/31.0% $P = 0.08$ Other CRC test in past year (% baseline/% followup): G1: 20.3%/27.5% G2: 19.6%/25.5% G3: 23.7%/21.1% G4: 26.4%/14.9% P = ns

CRC, colorectal cancer; FOBT, fecal occult blood test; LHA, lay health advisor; NR, not reported; ns, not significant; RCT, randomized controlled trial.

Outcomes for Chronic Disease Management

Chronic disease management: diabetes mellitus. *Study characteristics.* Four studies (eight articles; Table 25), three RCTs [27, 88-92, 124], and one prospective cohort study [93] examined outcomes of CHW interventions for diabetes care among underserved minority populations with type 2 diabetes mellitus. All studies were rated fair quality. Three studies [27, 88-93] used a high-intensity intervention; one study [124] used a moderate-intensity intervention.

Table 25. CHW chronic disease management: diabetes mellitus

Author, Year Study Design Population Setting Sample Size Quality	Intensity of CHW Intervention	Study Groups	Results
Beckham, 2008 [93] Cohort Health center for underserved with type 2 diabetes Hawaii N: 116 Fair	High	G1: Diabetes case management by CHW, including home visits, based on needs of patients; CHWs collaborate with multidisciplinary team to determine high-priority learning areas and develop an intervention plan to implement during subsequent visits, plan included a blood regimen and target levels, diet plan, exercise plan, medication schedule, insulin injection plan, and preventive health/health maintenance plan G2: Usual care with multidisciplinary team approach, minus CHW; glucose self-monitoring	HgbA1c, mean change from baseline (SD): G1: -2.2 (1.8) G2: -0.2 (1.5) $P < 0.0001$* *Note on P value: the investigators did not report a value comparing the groups; RTI researchers calculated the value using the data in the article
Corkery, 1997 [124] RCT Hispanic and African-American populations in East Harlem, New York City, New York N: 64 Fair	Moderate	G1: Intervention—CHW acted as liaison, attended clinic sessions, interpreted, reinforced self-care instructions and appointment reminders G2: Encounters occurred between nurse and patient only (control)	Diabetes education program completion: G1: 80% G2: 47% ($P = 0.01$) No difference in mean change in HgbA1c between groups
Gary 2000; [91] Batts 2001; [88] Gary 2003; [89] Vetter 2004; [92] Gary 2005 [90] RCT Project Sugar African-America	High High	G1: Usual care—continued on-going care from their own health professionals plus quarterly newsletter containing information on diabetes-related health topics G2: NCM intervention—RN + certified diabetes educator, 45- minute face-to-face clinic visits and/or telephone	HgbA1c, mean change from baseline at 2 years: G1: ref G2: -0.31 ± 0.49% G3: -0.30 ± 0.48% G4: 0.8 ± 0.52% ($P < 0.05$ for within-group change from baseline for G4 only)

Table 25. (Continued)

Author, Year Study Design Population Setting Sample Size Quality	Intensity of CHW Intervention	Study Groups	Results
population in East Baltimore, Maryland N: 186 Fair		contacts, direct patient care, management, education, counseling, followup, referral, physician feedback—goal was 3 visits per year G3: CHW intervention—45 to 60-minute face-to-face home visits and/or telephone contacts, no direct implementation of therapeutic strategies but facilitated preventive care by offering to schedule appointments and provide education, 3 visits per year G4: Combined NCM plus CHW—3 visits per year with each	LDL, mean change from baseline at 2 years: G1: -16.7± 5.5 mg/dl G2: +6 (approximate) (P < 0.05 for within-group change from baseline) G3: +6 (approximate) G4: +4 (approximate) (P < 0.05 for within-group change from baseline) SBP, mean change from baseline at 2 years: G1: ref G2: +6 (approximate) (P < 0.05 for within-group change from baseline) G3: -4 (approximate) G4: -2 (approximate) Dietary risk scores—validated, mean change from baseline at 2 years: G1: ref G2: -2.4 ± 1.99 G3: -3.45 ± 1.87 G4: -2.13 ± 1.92
Lujan, 2007 [27] RCT Mexican Americans in a major border city in Texas N: 150 Fair		G1: A team of 2 promotoras delivered 8 weekly, 2-hour participative group classes and followup to intervention group, using multiple audiovisual teaching aids and handouts, contacted class participants by telephone biweekly to answer questions, reinforce education, promoted behavior change, sent postcards biweekly G2: Usual care by clinic staff—verbal information and 1 or 2 pamphlets on diabetes self-management	HgbA1c at baseline (SD)/ 6 months (SD): G1: 8.21 (2.2)/7.76 (1.87) G2: 7.71 (1.49)/8.01 (1.8) Mean change between groups: P < 0.001 Bilingual Diabetes Knowledge Questionnaire (validated): baseline (SD)/6 months (SD): G1: 69.1 (13.6)/77.2 (14.4) G2: 66.9 (15.2)/65.1 (21.0) Mean change between groups: P <.002 Diabetes Health Belief Measure–(validated): baseline (SD)/6 months (SD): G1: 56.4 (12.2)/54.6 (8.4) G2: 57.0 (10.6)/50.8 (13.6) Mean change between groups: P < 0.01

Approx, approximately; CHW, Community Health Worker; DKQ, Diabetes Knowledge Questionnaire; HgbA1c, Hemoglobin A1c; LDL, low-density lipoprotein; NCM, nurse case manager; RCT, randomized controlled trial; RN, Registered nurse; SBP, systolic blood pressure.

The 6-month RCT conducted in Texas used a high-intensity intervention for Mexican Americans that compared eight weekly, 2-hour group classes with promotoras to usual care plus educational pamphlets [27]. The RCT in New York City used a moderate-intensity intervention for inner-city Hispanics and African Americans that evaluated the use of CHWs as clinic liaisons compared with nurse-patient encounters [124]. The Project Sugar trial RCT in Baltimore, Maryland, compared several high-intensity interventions in inner-city African

Americans with type 2 diabetes: (1) CHW face-to-face home visits and telephone contact, (2) nurse care manager intervention, (3) a combined nurse care manager and CHW, and (4) standard clinical care with an additional quarterly diabetes newsletter [88-92]. The prospective cohort study in Hawaii examined a high-intensity intervention comparing CHW diabetes case management, including home visits, in addition to a multidisciplinary team, with usual clinical care involving a multidisciplinary team approach [93]. Heterogeneity of population, study designs, interventions, and outcomes preclude quantitative synthesis of results.

Table 26. CHW chronic disease management: hypertension

Author, Year Study Design Population Setting Sample Size Quality	Intensity of CHW Intervention	Study Groups	Results
Levine, 2003 [98] RCT African Americans in inner-city Baltimore, Maryland N: 789 Fair	High	G1: G2 care plus 5 CHW visits with blood pressure measurement, addressing issues of blood pressure management and access to medical care G2: CHW home visit for education, counseling, and referral	Pre/postintervention blood pressure systolic/diastolic): G1: 147.7/89.2 (95% CI, 145.5-149.9/87.8-90.6) → 145/86.2 (95% CI, 142.3-147.7/84.2-88.2) G2: 148.6/89.3 (95% CI, 146.4-150.7/87.8-90.8) → 142.1/84.7 (95% CI, 138.8-145.4/82.7-86.7) $P < 0.05$ for differences between baseline and followup for each group, $P > 0.1$ between groups Percentage with adequate hypertension control (< 140/90): G1: 16% → 36% G2: 18% → 34% pre/post $P < 0.01$ group difference NS
Ward, 2000; [99]; Morisky, 2002 [23] RCT Inner-city African Americans and Hispanics	Moderate	G1: CHW post-clinic appointment counseling session G2: Appointment reminder cards and telephone calls	Percentage with blood pressure control (< 140/90)—baseline/ 6 months/12 months: G1: 35.2%/46%/46% ($P <$ 0.01) G2: 40.2%/42%/48% ($P <$ 0.01)
in a large West Coast city N: 1,367 Poor		G3: Home visits by CHW G4: Standard clinic care	G3: 29.7%/NR but "improved" G4: 36.9%/NR but "improved" All groups improved; differences between groups NR

Table 26. (Continued)

Author, Year Study Design Population Setting Sample Size Quality	Intensity of CHW Intervention	Study Groups	Results
Frate, 1983 [95] Frate, 1985 [94] Prospective cohort Rural central Mississippi N: 667 Poor	High	G1: Hypertension health counselors—monthly visits that encouraged compliance to both pharmacological and nonpharmacological therapy that had been prescribed G2: Family-based self-help G3: Church-based self-help	Proportion of hypertensives controlled (< 160/95): G1: 80.6% G2: 90.0% G3: 79.9% P (< 0.0001)
Bone, 1989 [123] Prospective cohort Low-income African Americans in emergency department in Baltimore, Maryland N: 722 Poor	Moderate	G1: Control (not able to be contacted by CHW) G2: Contacted by CHW; initially, all patients contacted by CHWs in emergency department; CHWs measured pulse and blood pressure, provided educational counseling, identified barriers related to referrals, assisted with appointment-keeping and adherence to treatment plan; session lasted about 20 minutes	Returned to emergency department for followup appointment: G1: 41% G2: 60% ($P < 0.001$)

CHW, community health worker; NS, not significant; RCT, randomized controlled trial.

Overview of results. Of these four studies on diabetes management, two studies found the CHW intervention to be beneficial in decreasing hemoglobin A1c (HgbA1c) as compared with usual care; [27, 93] conversely, two studies found no difference between groups in mean change from baseline in HgbA1c [88-92, 124]. The Texas study also evaluated outcomes of knowledge and found that the CHW intervention was effective compared with usual clinical care in increasing diabetes knowledge [27]. The Hawaii study found that diabetes case management by a CHW in conjunction with a multidisciplinary team was more effective at decreasing HgbA1c than a multidisciplinary team alone [93]. The New York study demonstrated that a CHW liaison was more effective than usual clinical care in behavioral changes leading to program completion rates [124]. Project Sugar, a high-intensity study, found significant changes from baseline within, but not between, groups for various health outcomes [88-92].

Knowledge. The Texas study evaluated outcomes for improved knowledge at 6 months in diabetic patients following eight weekly CHW-led group classes in Mexican Americans [27]. A validated tool, the bilingual Diabetes Knowledge Questionnaire (DKQ), showed a difference between arms, with an improved score in the CHW group compared with the group receiving usual care plus educational pamphlets ($P < 0.002$) [27].

Behavior. Project Sugar evaluated dietary risk scores (which identifies positive as well as problematic dietary behaviors and measures potential barriers to dietary change). Scores improved across all CHW arms as compared with the usual clinical care group following a high- intensity CHW intervention (all CHW arms versus usual clinical care [score ± standard deviation]: -2.4 ± 1.99 versus -3.45 ± 1.87 versus -2.13 ± 1.92; *P* not reported) [88-92]. The New York study demonstrated an increased proportion of completion of a diabetes education program after a low-intensity CHW intervention compared with usual clinical care (80 percent versus 47 percent, $P = 0.01$) [124].

Satisfaction. No study reported outcomes about satisfaction with diabetes care.

Health outcomes. The Texas trial demonstrated better improvement in diabetes control (measured by mean change in HgbA1c) in the high-intensity CHW intervention group than in the usual care group after 6 months ($P < 0.001$) [27]. The Hawaii study found that a high-intensity CHW intervention in conjunction with a multidisciplinary team was more effective in decreasing mean HgbA1c when compared with usual care with a multidisciplinary team (-2.2 versus 0.2) [93]. The Hawaii study investigators did not report *P* value comparing the groups; we were able to calculate it using the data provided in the article and found the difference to be statistically significant ($P < 0.0001$) [93]. Project Sugar reported no significant change between the four study groups for the primary outcome, HgbA1c. The only group with a significant improvement from baseline to2 years was the CHW plus nurse care manager arm (improvement of 0.8 percent ± 0.52 percent, $P < 0.05$) [88-92]. Postintervention, a power calculation showed the study was powered to detect a difference of only 1.2 percent change in HgbA1c. Secondary outcomes from Project Sugar included low density lipoprotein (LDL) cholesterol, systolic blood pressure, and diastolic blood pressure; none differed significantly between study groups in change from baseline measures. LDL cholesterol changed for the worse within the CHW plus nurse care manager arm (+4 mg/dl, $P < 0.05$) [88-92].

Health care utilization. No study evaluated diabetes care utilization.

Chronic disease management: hypertension. *Study characteristics.* Four studies (five articles; Table 26), two RCTs [23, 98, 99] and two prospective cohorts [94, 95, 123], examined outcomes of moderate-intensity CHW interventions for blood pressure management among adult patients with hypertension. We rated one study as fair quality and three as poor quality. All four studies evaluated a CHW intervention compared with an intervention that involved a CHW in a lesser capacity [23, 94, 95, 98, 99, 123]. The two RCTs, one fair [98] and one poor [99] quality, evaluated CHW interventions in inner-city minority populations [23, 98, 99].

The fair-quality trial from Baltimore, Maryland, evaluated a CHW home visit for patient education, counseling, and referral compared with a CHW home visit plus five additional visits for blood pressure measurement and management, and access to medical care [98]. The poor-quality RCT from the West Coast, rated as such because of a high attrition rate, use of a completers analysis, and high potential for bias, evaluated CHW postclinic appointment counseling sessions, CHW home visits, appointment reminder cards and calls, and standard clinical care [23, 99].

The prospective cohort study from rural central Mississippi, which we rated as poor quality because of a high potential for confounding and inappropriate statistical methods, evaluated a moderate-intensity CHW intervention using CHWs as "hypertension health counselors" in providing monthly visits encouraging compliance with previously prescribed pharmacological and nonpharmacological therapies [94, 95]. The other prospective cohort study from Baltimore, Maryland, which we rated poor because of a lack of methods describing an analysis plan a priori, a high potential for confounding, and lack of comparison of participant characteristics at baseline, evaluated a moderate-intensity CHW intervention [123]. It examined the impact on appointment followup of a CHW followup telephone call after an emergency department visit during which patients had their blood pressure measured, were provided education counseling, and were assisted with appointment keeping and adherence to a treatment plan. The comparison group included patients who had received a single CHW visit in the emergency department but who could not be reached later for assistance in appointment keeping [123]. Heterogeneity of study designs, interventions, and outcomes preclude quantitative synthesis of results.

Overview of results. We did not find any fair- or good-quality studies that compared the impact of a CHW intervention with usual care on blood pressure control. Of the three studies that evaluated blood pressure control, only the Mississippi prospective cohort demonstrated a significant difference between study groups in terms of proportion of hypertensive subjects controlled (defined in this study as blood pressure less than 160/95) [94, 95]. Neither RCT demonstrated between-group differences in blood pressure control [23, 98, 99]. However, these studies did note improvement from baseline to study completion within all groups, some of which were statistically significant [23, 98, 99]. The Baltimore prospective cohort did not evaluate blood pressure control but instead examined health care utilization [123]. This study demonstrated that CHW worker followup was more effective than no followup in increasing return visit appointment rates.

Knowledge. No study reported improved knowledge.

Behavior. No study reported improved behaviors.

Satisfaction. No study reported satisfaction outcomes.

Health outcomes. We did not find any fair- or good-quality studies that compared the impact of a CHW intervention with usual care on blood pressure control. Three of the four studies did report on blood pressure control. Both RCTs found an improvement within most groups but no difference between groups in terms of blood pressure control [23, 98, 99]. The fair-quality RCT demonstrated that the low-intensity CHW arm (1 home visit) and the high-intensity CHW arm (6 home visits) both improved blood pressure control. However, the difference between the groups was not statistically significant [98]. The poor-quality RCT also demonstrated an improvement in blood pressure within all groups, including the usual care arm, but no significant difference between groups [23, 99]. The Mississippi prospective cohort study did not report statistical tests for either between- or within-group comparisons [94].

Health care utilization. The poor-quality prospective cohort in a Baltimore emergency department demonstrated that patients in the low-intensity CHW intervention were more likely to return for a followup appointment than were patients in the comparison group (60 percent versus 40 percent, $P < 0.001$) [123]. However, the comparison patients were not able to be contacted for followup by the CHW, thus biasing the results for this outcome in favor of the intervention arm [123].

Chronic disease management: infectious diseases. *Study characteristics.* One RCT of fair quality examined outcomes of a CHW intervention to facilitate access to health care for tuberculosis (TB) in a homeless population with positive purified protein derivative (PPD) test results in San Francisco, California (Table 27) [122]. This study used a moderate-intensity model. CHWs who were familiar with homelessness were assigned to TB-infected individuals and responsible for accompanying them to their clinic appointments [122]. Outcomes were compared with outcomes for a group receiving a monetary incentive to attend the TB clinic in addition to an appointment and bus tokens and with a control group who were given clinic appointments and bus tokens.

Overview of results. This RCT demonstrated that a CHW intervention was less effective than the monetary incentive but more effective than usual care in leading to adherence to a first followup appointment [122].

Knowledge. This RCT did not report outcomes for improved knowledge.

Behavior. This RCT did not report outcomes for improved behaviors.

Satisfaction. This RCT did not report outcomes of satisfaction.

Health outcomes. This RCT did not report outcomes of health.

Health care utilization. A moderate-intensity CHW intervention was less effective than a monetary incentive ($5) in increasing adherence to a first followup clinic appointment (75 percent [95% CI, 70-80] versus 84 percent [95% CI, 76-92], P = not reported). However, the CHW intervention was more effective than a control group who received an appointment and bus tokens (75 percent [95% CI, 70-80] versus 53 percent [95% CI, 47-59], $P = 0.004$) [122].

Chronic disease management: back pain. *Study characteristics.* One RCT of fair quality evaluated a moderate-intensity intervention of four 2-hour weekly group classes led by CHWs compared with usual care supplemented by a book on back pain (Table 28) [114]. The classes focused on applying problem-solving techniques for back pain self-management and included educational materials (book and videos) supporting active management of back pain [114].

Overview of results. This fair-quality RCT found that a moderate-intensity CHW intervention was significantly effective in reducing back pain when compared with a control group at 6 months; the groups did not differ significantly at 12 months [114].

Knowledge. This RCT did not report outcomes for improved knowledge.

Table 27. CHW chronic disease management: infectious diseases

Author, Year Study Design Population Setting Sample Size Quality	Intensity of CHW Intervention	Study Groups	Results
Pilote, 1996 [122] RCT Homeless people with positive purified protein deriviative for tuberculosis in San Francisco, California N = 244 Fair	Moderate	G1: Peer health advisor—met with patient and took them to clinic appointment, facilitated paperwork, reviewed physician recommendations G2: Monetary incentive—$5 at clinic, appointment, and bus tokens G3: Usual care—appointment and bus tokens	Adherence to first followup appointment (95% CI): P calculated vs. G3 G1: 75% (70-80); ($P = 0.004$) G2: 84% (76-92); ($P < 0.001$) G3: 53% (47-59)

CI, confidence interval; RCT, randomized controlled trial.

Table 28. CHW chronic disease management: back pain

Author, Year Study Design Population Setting Sample Size Quality	Intensity of CHW Intervention	Study Groups	Results
Von Korff, 1998 [114] RCT People with chronic back pain in Washington state N = 255 Fair	Moderate	G1: 4, 2-hour classes held once a week, with 10 to 15 participants, led by 2 CHWs G2: Usual care includes back pain book	"The next time I have back or leg pain, I will try to manage the problem without seeing a health professional" (not validated): G1: 77% agreed G2: 60% agreed ($P = 0.008$) 50% or greater reduction in Roland Disability Questionnaire Score from baseline at 6 months (validated): G1: 47.9% G2: 33% ($P = 0.02$) Roland Disability at 12 months (validated): G1: 5.75 (6.31) G2: 6.75 (6.39) ($P = 0.092$) Worry rating (0-10) at 12 months (not validated): G1: 2.63 (2.58) G2: 3.83 (3.08) ($P = 0.013$)

CHW, community health worker; RCT, randomized controlled trial.

Behavior. This RCT did not report changes in participant behavior.

Satisfaction. This RCT did not report outcomes of satisfaction.

Health outcomes. The moderate-intensity CHW intervention was more effective in decreasing participant back pain than usual care supplemented by a book on back pain at 6 months [114]. More participants in the intervention arm achieved a 50 percent or greater reduction in Roland Disability Score from baseline than in the control group at 6 months (47.9 percent versus 33 percent, $P = 0.02$) [114]. However, Roland Disability Scores at 12 months did not differ between arms (5.75 ± 6.31 versus 6.75 ±6.39, $P = 0.092$) [114]. The authors attributed this lack of difference to the fact that the intervention was intended not to reduce pain intensity but rather to lower patient worries about back pain [114]. Additionally, participants receiving a CHW intervention had a lower worry rating (unvalidated tool) than those in the control group at 12 months (2.63 ± 2.58 versus 3.83 ± 3.08, $P = 0.013$) [114].

Health care utilization. This RCT did not report on health care utilization.

Other. Participants in the CHW arm reported being more likely to self-manage back or leg pain than those in the control arm, a measure of self-efficacy (77 percent versus 60 percent, $P = 0.008$) [114].**gement: mental health.** *Study characteristics.* One RCT of poor quality with three trial arms evaluated an assertive community treatment with a CHW intervention compared with an assertive community treatment alone and with a brokered case management intervention (Table 29) [120, 121]. The study population included people in St. Louis, Missouri, who were homeless or at risk for being homeless and were diagnosed with erious psychiatric diagnoses [120, 121]. The CHWs' role was to assist with daily living and be available for leisure activities. This intervention was rated as high-intensity as defined in KQ 1. A high rate of attrition (only 85 of 165 provided followup) contributed to the poor-quality rating of this study [120, 121].

Overview of results. Clients in the assertive community treatment arm plus a CHW did not differ in results when compared with the assertive community treatment group alone, although for many outcomes both of these arms were superior to the brokered case management arm [120, 121]. The assertive community treatment arms (both with and without a CHW) had more contact with their case managers and were more satisfied than those in the brokered case management arm [120, 121]. Clients in the assertive community treatment also had fewer psychiatric symptoms at 18 months than clients in the brokered condition [120, 121]. Days in stable housing did not differ among groups [120, 121].

Knowledge. This RCT did not report outcomes for improved knowledge.

Behavior. This RCT did not report outcomes for improved behaviors.

Table 29. CHW chronic disease management: mental health

Author, Year Study Design Population Setting Sample Size Quality	Intensity of CHW Intervention	Study Groups	Results
Wolff, 1997 [121] Morse, 1997 [120] RCT Homeless with serious psychiatric conditions in St. Louis, Missouri N = 165 Poor	High	G1: Assertive community treatment—intensive individualized treatment, responsibility for providing or coordinating all services needed by client, persistent followup and in-person service delivery, performed by staff with backgrounds in psychology, social work, and counseling G2: G1 plus CHW, whose role was to assist with activities of daily living and be available for leisure activities G3: Brokered case management	Number of days in stable housing in past month—baseline (SD)/18 months (SD): G1: 6.36 (11.71)/21.75 (12.76) G2: 4.94 (11.08)/17.54 (14.45) G3: 7.18 (12.38)/16.00 (14.86) ($P < 0.31$) Client satisfaction (validated): G1: 3.27 (0.42) G2: 3.12 (0.57) G3: 2.74 (0.68) $P < 0.01$ Brief Psychiatric Rating Scale Total Symptom Score (validated): G1: 53.54 (15.54)/39.96 (12.25) G2: 57.97 (20.29)/38.77 (12.23) G3: 50.6 (14/31)/51.6 (16.7) $P = 0.001$ Program contact (days/month): G1: 8.29 (7.51) G2: 6.95 (4.91) G3: 0.3 (0.49) $P < 0.001$

CHW: community health worker; RCT, randomized controlled trial; SD: standard deviation.

Satisfaction. Clients in the assertive community treatment arms (both with and without a CHW) were more satisfied with their treatment program than clients in the brokered case management arm (satisfaction score ± standard deviation: 3.12 ± 0.57 versus 3.27 ± 0.42 versus 2.74 ± 0.68, $P < 0.05$) [120, 121].

Health outcomes. Clients in the assertive community treatment arm plus a CHW did not differ in health outcome results as compared with the assertive community treatment group alone. Clients in the assertive community treatment arms (both with and without a CHW) had fewer psychiatric symptoms as rated by the Brief Psychiatric Rating Scale (BPRS) at 18 months compared to baseline than did those in the brokered case management arm (baseline (SD)/18- month followup (SD): 57.97 (20.29)/38.77 (12.23) versus 53.54 (15.54)/39.96 (12.25) versus 50.60 (14.31)/51.60 (16.70), $P = 0.001$ for any difference among the three groups; P for comparison of either assertive community treatment arm not reported) [120, 121]. Days in stable housing between groups did not differ across the groups.

Health care utilization. Use of health services did not differ between the assertive community treatment plus a CHW arm and the assertive community treatment group alone. Clients in the assertive community treatment arms (both with and without a CHW) had more days in contact with the program than did clients in the brokered case management arm (6.95 (4.91) versus 8.29 (7.51) versus 0.3 (0.49), $P < 0.05$).

Chronic disease management: asthma. *Study characteristics.* Two RCTs (three articles), one good-quality [96, 97], and one fair-quality [100], examined outcomes of CHW interventions for asthma care among pediatric patients with persistent asthma. Both studies used a highly resource-intensive CHW model. Both studies provided comprehensive multifaceted interventions that included an environmental assessment, asthma action plan, education, referrals, allergy control mattress covers and pillows, vacuums, and cleaning supplies, pest management, and smoking cessation assistance to the high-intensity intervention arm, delivered over a year in several home visits. The Seattle King County Healthy Homes (SKCHH) project (Washington State) compared outcomes for children receiving a high-intensity multivisit home intervention with those for children receiving a low-intensity single home visit that included an environmental assessment, some education, and bedding encasements, followed by the full intervention after a year [96, 97]. The Community Action Against Asthma (CAAA) project adapted the SKCHH project to Detroit, Michigan, comparing a group receiving the high-intensity multivisit home intervention with a control group receiving an asthma information booklet and the full intervention after a year [100] Variations in measures of health behavior, outcomes, and health care utilization preclude quantitative synthesis of the results.

Overview of results. Two trials demonstrated that high-intensity CHW interventions are more effective than either low-intensity interventions or a control group in reducing unscheduled use of health care services and improving psychological outcomes for caregivers. Both studies demonstrated changes in behavior, such as increased use of bed encasements and vacuuming, associated with the materials distributed by the CHW, but not for other behaviors that may have required external or additional resources or change, such as removal of mold or reduced exposure to environmental tobacco smoke. Both studies demonstrated significant improvements within but not across trial arms for some measures of symptoms [96, 97, 100], reduced days with activity limitations, and reduced use of beta-agonists [96, 97]. Authors postulated that these results could be explained either because a minimal intervention may be effective for some outcomes or because of regression to the mean, temporal trends, or the Hawthorne effect (improvement in performance attributable to being observed) among the less intensive or control group participants [96, 97]. Nevertheless, for health outcomes demonstrating a difference between trial arms such as symptom days, the more intense arm was more effective than the less intense or control arm.

Knowledge. Neither study reported outcomes for improved knowledge of asthma triggers.

Table 30. CHW asthma interventions and behavior

Author, Year Population Setting Sample Size Quality	Intensity of CHW Intervention	Study Groups	Results
Krieger et al., 2005; [96] Krieger et al., 2002 [97] RCT Children ages 4-12 years with persistent asthma Low-income households in King County, Washington N: 274 Good	High	G1: Environmental assessment; asthma action plan; education and social support; mattress covers, pillows, vacuum, cleaning supplies; smoking cessation referral; 4-8 visits over 12 months G2: Environmental home assessment action plan, limited education, bedding encasements; full intervention after 12 months	Behavior, summary score of trigger reduction behaviors Across groups comparison: GEE coefficient (95% CI, 0.41 (-0.13-0.95); *P* = 0.141) Frequencies of actions to reduce dust exposure and the use of bedding encasements increased more in the high-intensity group; kitchen ventilation improved more in the low-intensity group. Neither group increased the frequency of washing sheets or dusting, nor reduced exposure to pets (although pet ownership was uncommon among participants) and smoking in the home; behavior summary score improved in both groups, and the across-group difference was not significant
Parker et al., 2008 [100] RCT Children ages 7-11 years with persistent asthma Southwest and eastside Detroit, Michigan N: 298 Fair	High	G1: Environmental assessment; asthma action plan based on allergy tests; education and social support; mattress covers, pillows, vacuum, cleaning supplies; counseling on environmental tobacco smoke; integrated pest management services; minimum 9 planned home visits over 12 months G2: Asthma information booklet, full intervention after 12 months	Intervention effect (or-intervention/or-control) Vacuum cleaner used: 29.5 (6.90, 126); $P < 0.0001$ Allergen cover on child's pillow: 19.7 (4.12, 94.2); $P = 0.0006$ Allergen cover on child's mattress: 9.70 (4.33, 21.7); $P < 0.0001$ Visible mold growth removed: 0.74 (0.33, 1.66); $P = 0.47$ Child is around people who smoke: 0.60 (0.28, 1.32); $P = 0.20$ Statistically significant intervention effect in the reduction of concentration of dog allergen per gram of bedroom dust ($P < 0.001$) but not for cockroach, dust mite, or cat allergen concentration

CI, confidence interval; GEE, generalized estimating equation; RCT, randomized controlled trial.

Behavior. Both studies examined a variety of behavioral changes (Table 30). Both studies reported increased use of materials provided—that is, mattress covers, pillows, and vacuums, suggesting reduced exposure to dust mites— in the more intense arm. Both studies failed to find differences between the two arms for behavioral changes associated with smoking cessation. Other behaviors that did not differ between arms included removal of pets and use of exhaust fans in the bathroom [96, 97] and removal of mold [100].

Satisfaction. Neither study reported outcomes for satisfaction.

Health outcomes. The SKCHH project reported on the number of symptom days in the past 2 weeks. The CAAA project looked at the occurrence of more than 2 symptom days per week for children not on any controller medication or corticosteroids (Table 31).

Table 31. CHW asthma interventions and health outcomes

Author, Year Study Design Population Setting Sample Size Quality	Intensity of CHW Intervention	Study Groups	Results
Krieger et al., 2005; [96] Krieger et al., 2002 [97] RCT Children ages 4-12 years with persistent asthma Low-income households in King County, Washington N: 274 Good	High	G1: Environmental assessment; asthma action plan; education and social support; mattress covers, pillows, vacuum, cleaning supplies; smoking cessation referral; 4-8 visits over 12 months G2: Environmental home assessment action plan; limited education; bedding encasements; full intervention after 12 months	Pediatric Asthma Caregiver QoL Scale (score range 1-7 with higher scores indicating better QoL) Score at exit (G1 vs. G2): 5.6 vs. 5.4 GEE coefficient 0.58 (95% CI, 0.18-0.99), *P* = 0.005; NNT = 4.8 ITT analysis yielded similar results: improvements in QoL were greater in G1 (data NR, *P* = 0.009) Asthma symptom days (self-reported number of 24-hour periods during 2 weeks before interview with asthma symptoms: wheezing, tightness in chest, cough, shortness of breath, slowing down activities due to asthma, nighttime awakenings): G1 vs. G2 at exit: 3.2 vs. 3.9 GEE coefficient -1.24 (95% CI, -2.9 to 0.4), *P* = 0.138 Days with activity limitation over 2-week period Score at exit (G1 vs. G2): 1.5 vs. 1.7 GEE coefficient -1.5 (95% CI, -2.84 to -0.15), OR, 0.22 (0.06, 0.86), P = 0.29 Missed school in past 2 weeks: G1 vs. G2 at exit: 12.2% vs. 20.3% GEE coefficient -0.77 (95% CI, -1.70 to 0.16), OR, 0.46 (0.18, 1.18), *P* = 0.105 Days used controller medication over 2–week period: G1 vs. G2 at exit: 3.5 vs. 3.6 GEE coefficient -1.03 (95% CI, -2.79 to 0.73), *P* = 0.250 Days used beta2-agonist over 2-week period: G1 vs. G2 at exit: 4.0 vs. 4.0 GEE coefficient -0.23 (95% CI, -1.88 to 1.42), *P* = 0.781 Caregiver missed work in past 2 weeks: G1 vs. G2 at exit: 11.2% vs. 13.0% GEE coefficient 0.07 (95% CI, -0.91 to 1.0.5), OR, 1.07 (0.40, 2.85), *P* = 0.890

Author, Year Study Design Population Setting Sample Size Quality	Intensity of CHW Intervention	Study Groups	Results
Parker et al., 2008 [100] RCT Children ages 7-11 years with persistent asthma Southwest and eastside Detroit, Michigan N: 298 Fair	High	G1: Environmental assessment; asthma action plan based on allergy tests; education and social support; mattress covers, pillows, vacuum, cleaning supplies; counseling on environmental tobacco smoke; integrated pest management services; minimum 9 planned home visits over 12 months G2: Asthma information booklet, full intervention after 12 months	Caregiver depressive symptoms measured by Center for Epidemiologic Studies Depression Scale (CES-D) mean at baseline/endpoint: G1: 1.62/1.54 G2: 1.58/1.64 $P = 0.0218$ Improvements in both instrumental and emotional social support combined and instrumental support alone were not statistically significant (data NR) Child's self-reported average asthma symptom frequency: G1: symptoms occurred less frequently at baseline for all 8 symptoms assessed G2: symptoms occurred less frequently for 6 of 8 symptoms Persistent cough at baseline, postintervention (on a 6-point scale, higher is worse): G1: 3.81, 3.36 G2: 3.48, 3.44 $P = 0.034$ Cough with exercise at baseline, postintervention (on a 6-point scale, higher is worse): G1: 4.27, 3.69 G2: 3.80, 3.66 $P = 0.017$ Has any symptom more than 2 days per week and not on a corticosteroid G1 (pre/post) vs. G2 (pre/post) intervention effect (95% CI): 60/42 vs. 51/46; 0.56 (0.29 to 1.06); $P = 0.073$ Has any symptom more than 2 days per week and not on any controller G1 (pre/post) vs. G2 (pre/post) intervention effect (95% CI): 53/32 vs. 38/37; 0.39 (0.20 to 0.73); $P = 0.004$

CI, confidence interval; GEE, generalized estimating equation; ITT, intention to treat; NNT, number needed to treated; NR, not reported; OR, odds ratio; QoL, quality of life; vs., versus.

Results from these two trials were mixed. The Seattle (SKCHH) project reported nonsignificant differences between the arms in the reduction in symptoms days, whereas the Detroit (CAAA) project found significant differences between the trial arms for children not on any controller medication (OR, 0.39 [95 percent CI, 0.20-0.73]) [96, 97]. The differences between trial arms in reduction of symptom days was not statistically significant in the subset of children not on corticosteroids [100].

Table 32. CHW asthma interventions and health care utilization

Author, Year Population Setting Sample Size Quality	Intensity of CHW Intervention	Study Groups	Results
Krieger et al., 2005; [96] Krieger et al., 2002 [97] Children ages 4-12 years with persistent asthma Low-income households in King County, Washington N: 274 Good	High	G1: Environmental assessment; asthma action plan; education and social support; mattress covers, pillows, vacuum, cleaning supplies; smoking cessation referral; 4 to 8 visits over 12 months G2: Environmental home assessment action plan, limited education, bedding encasements; full intervention after 12 months	Urgent health services used over 2 months G1 vs. G2 at exit: 8.4% vs. 16.4% GEE coefficient -0.97 (95% CI, -1.8 to -0.12), OR 0.38 (0.16, 0.89), P = 0.026; NNT = 12.9 ITT analysis yielded similar results: improvements in urgent health services were greater in G1 (data NR, P = 0.062)
Parker et al., 2008 [100] Children ages 7-11 years with persistent asthma Southwest and eastside Detroit, Michigan N: 298 Fair	High	G1: Environmental assessment; asthma action plan based on allergy tests; education and social support; mattress covers, pillows, vacuum, cleaning supplies; counseling on environmental tobacco smoke; integrated pest management services; minimum 9 planned home visits over 12 months G2: Asthma information booklet, full intervention after 12 months	Reduction in unscheduled health care utilization for asthma Percentage needed unscheduled medical care–G1 (pre/post) vs. G2 (pre/post); intervention effect (95% CI): In past 3 months: 50/45 vs. 42/56; 0.43 (0.23 to 0.80); P = 0.007 In past 12 months: 65/59 vs. 58/73; 0.40 (0.22 to 0.74); P = 0.004

CI; confidence interval; GEE, generalized estimating equation; ITT, intention to treat; NNT, number not treated; NR, not reported; OR, odds ratio; RCT, randomized controlled trial.

The Seattle (SKCHH) project also examined differences in trial arms in days with activity limitation, use of beta-agonists, use of controller medications, missed school days for the child, and missed caregiver workdays. With the exception of days with activity limitations, the study found no differences between the intervention arms [96, 97]. It also found a significantly higher increase in caregiver quality of life (measured by the Center for Epidemiologic Studies Depression Scale in the more intense arm (coefficient for difference between groups in mean change from exit to baseline: 0.58 [95 percent CI, 0.18-0.99]) [96, 97].

The Detroit (CAAA) project found significant improvements in symptoms for both intervention and control arms, but differences were statistically significant only for coughing with exercise and persistent cough. It also found significant differences between trial arms in some but not all measures of lung function; these results could potentially be explained by seasonal influences, changes in instrumentation, and inadequate power [100]. Finally, it reported a statistically significant reduction ($P = 0.0218$) in caregiver depressive symptoms (measured by the Center for Epidemiologic Studies Depression Scale) in the intervention arm (mean value at baseline and followup: 1.62 and 1.54) compared to a rise in depressive symptoms in the control arm (mean value at baseline and followup: 1.58 to 1.64). The study found no statistically significant differences between the two groups in changes in social support between baseline and the endpoint [100].

Health care utilization. Both studies (Table 32). found a significant difference in the reduction in unscheduled medical care—emergency room visits, hospitalizations, and unscheduled doctor visits—favoring the more intense intervention at three points: 2 months (OR: 0.38; 95% CI, 0.16-0.89) [96, 97], 3 months (OR: 0.43; 95% CI, 0.23-0.80) [100], and 12 months (OR: 0.40; 95% CI, 0.22-0.74) [100].

KQ 3: Cost-Effectiveness of Community Health Worker Interventions

Overview of Economic Analyses

A total of nine studies that met inclusion criteria for this review contained information about intervention costs, cost-effectiveness, or cost-benefits. We focused here on the six studies that also demonstrated effectiveness of the CHW intervention, either as compared with the alternatives that were analyzed or as compared with baseline, or usual, care [17-22, 75, 80, 96, 104, 121]. The studies on CHWs that included economic information varied a great deal in terms of the populations targeted for intervention, the types of interventions implemented and the settings for those interventions, the alternatives that were analyzed, and the outcomes the interventions sought to impact.

Targeted populations, for example, ranged from Latina women to low-income infants and children. The types of interventions using CHWs as a study arm included early childhood and child health interventions, cancer screening interventions, and chronic disease management interventions. Some studies evaluated alternatives that varied intensity levels for the CHW intervention; others compared the CHW intervention without nurse-delivered interventions; and others compared the CHW intervention with lower intensity alternatives that did not involve direct interaction with targeted patients (e.g., providing written materials only). Study outcomes also varied a great deal across studies, reflecting the diversity of types of interventions and targeted populations (e.g., outcomes related to use of health care, child health and development, and impacts on usual activities such as work or school). Intervention settings also varied; some CHW interventions focused on working with participants in their homes, one focused on working with homeless individuals, and another took place in urban churches.

The three studies with economic information that we eventually excluded involved (1) a diet change intervention that targeted Hispanic women [64], (2) an environmental tobacco smoke intervention that targeted young Latino children [67], and (3) a children's immunization intervention that compared CHW interventions with mail or telephone interventions for raising children's immunization rates [69, 70]. These three studies produced no statistically significant impact on CHW intervention groups as compared with outcomes in the control groups.

In the discussion below, we cite only the articles with data specific to the cost-analysis; studies spanned several other citations specific to outcomes not relevant to the discussion below.

Economics: cancer screening. *Study characteristics.* Two studies (one trial and one prospective cohort) evaluated program costs or cost-effectiveness for CHW interventions that sought to improve women's mammography rates [17, 22]. The ROSE study targeted low-income, rural white, African-American, and Native-American women in North Carolina ages 40 years and older, all of whom had not had a mammogram in the previous 12 months [17, 18]. These women were randomly assigned to a high-intensity CHW intervention, which involved three home visits with followup telephone calls and mailings, or to a comparison group. The CHW intervention was delivered for a period of 12 to 14 months. The LAMP CHW study collected data on program costs and cost-effectiveness for a low-intensity cancer screening CHW intervention [19-22, 104]. The intervention was a church-based telephone counseling program that targeted female church members ages 50 to 80 years to promote mammography. Some of these women had obtained mammograms 1 to 2 years before the initial survey and within the 2-year window before that ("adherent" group), whereas others had not ("nonadherent" group). Church volunteers made one telephone call per 12-month period to encourage and address barriers to mammography.

Overview of economic analysis results. Both studies report program costs and the costs per additional mammography screening [17, 22]. Both studies estimated program costs using a program or funder perspective (i.e., including only those costs that would be incurred by a prevention program to deliver the intervention); that is, they did not employ a societal perspective. Because the LAMP study used volunteer labor, the costs of the intervention from the program perspective are necessarily low compared with the costs of the ROSE intervention, which paid their CHWs. To better understand what costs would be if CHWs had to be hired to deliver the LAMP intervention, Stockdale et al. [22] also report two alternative program cost estimates—one that values volunteer time at the minimum wage and another that values volunteer time at the average wage rate.

Measures of effectiveness for economic analysis. The main effectiveness outcome that both studies used for their economic analyses was mammogram receipt in the 12 months before a followup survey. The ROSE study outcomes were based on review of a woman's medical record [17, 22]. The LAMP study outcomes were based on participants' self-reports via a telephone interview; it also estimated life-years saved based on a model of screening, diagnosis, and treatment for breast cancer [22].

Economic outcomes. The total cost of the ROSE intervention was estimated to be $329,054 [17], which translates to approximately $404 per participant, based on the 815 participants who fully participated in the intervention and data collection. The year of costs was not reported for the ROSE study. Program costs for the LAMP intervention were estimated to be $11 per participant in 1997 dollars when the opportunity cost of CHW volunteers' time was excluded from the cost calculation. Costs were estimated at $28 per person when CHW volunteers' time was valued at the minimum wage and $52 per person when an average wage rate for each type of volunteer was used (1997 dollars) [22]. To compare ROSE and LAMP costs, we assumed that the ROSE costs are in 2000 dollars (the midpoint of the study time period, 1998 through 2002). Using the consumer price index for all urban consumers (CPI-U) to adjust the LAMP intervention cost of $52 per participant in 1997 dollars to 2000 dollars yields an estimate of $56 per LAMP participant, as contrasted with the high-intensity ROSE intervention cost of about $404 per participant.

Both studies also reported costs per additional screening [17, 22]. Paskett et al. estimated the impact of the ROSE intervention to be 66 additional mammograms in the CHW intervention group, resulting in a cost-effectiveness ratio of $4,986 per additional mammogram (assumed 2000 dollars) [17]. Stockdale et al. estimated the impact of the LAMP intervention to be 3.24 additional mammography screenings for each of the 45 churches that participated in the study, resulting in an estimated cost per additional screening of $903 (1997 dollars) when CHW volunteers' time was valued at the average wage rate [22]. Although these findings appear to suggest that the LAMP intervention had a much lower cost per additional mammogram received than did the ROSE intervention, the effectiveness and cost-effectiveness results are not comparable between these two studies because the LAMP intervention targeted women who were both adherent and nonadherent with screening guidelines, whereas the ROSE intervention targeted only nonadherent women. Focusing on results for the nonadherent LAMP participants only, the estimated intervention effectiveness is 1.46 additional screenings per church per year (not statistically significant), which we estimate to produce a cost-effectiveness ratio of $2,005 per additional mammography screening in 1997 dollars, or $2,151 in 2000 dollars, when the time of CHWs is valued using expected wage rates.

Stockdale et al. also estimated the cost per life-year saved by the LAMP intervention and subsequent mammography screening as $46,308 (1997 dollars) [22], when CHW time was valued using expected wage rates ($33,632 plus the estimated cost per life-year saved for mammography screening of $12,676).

Economics: chronic disease management. *Study characteristics.* Two studies provided economic information on the management of chronic diseases; both studies are described in more detail in the last section of KQ 2. One study evaluated an asthma control intervention for children; [96] the other evaluated an intervention to prevent homelessness in patients with mental illness [121].

The asthma intervention, known as the Seattle King County Healthy Homes (SKCHH) project, evaluated a 1-year high-intensity CHW intervention approach, involving five to nine CHW home visits [96]. The investigators compared this high-intensity intervention with a low- intensity version that involved only one CHW home visit and evaluated health care utilization and costs for participants, intervention program costs, and other measures related to asthma control, quality of life, and productivity.

The homelessness prevention intervention compared three alternative case management approaches for people with mental illness at high risk of homelessness:

- brokered case management—a low-intensity intervention that can be viewed as the baseline, or usual care, approach;

- assertive community treatment—a high-intensity intervention that involves frequent interaction with the client and assistance with a host of activities and social service acquisition; and
- assertive community treatment with CHWs—a high-intensity CHW intervention that consists of assertive community treatment, adding a CHW to interact with and assist clients [121].

Each intervention was provided over 18 months. Key outcomes were health care and social services utilization, program costs, and pre- and postintervention measures of 6 months of costs for health care and social services among study participants.

Overview of economic analysis results. Both studies report program costs per participant from the program perspective. For the Seattle study, Krieger et al. [96] estimated the cost of the 12- month intervention by summing payments for salary and fringe benefits, supplies, rent, travel, and office expenses and adding indirect costs of 13 percent. For the homelessness prevention study, Wolff et al. [121] estimated the additional intervention program costs of assertive community treatment, with and without CHWs, as the costs above those for brokered case management; their estimates values CHW time at the minimum wage.

Both studies estimated the impact of the intervention on health care and/or social services costs for program participants. For example, Krieger et al. assessed the pre- and postintervention costs of urgent care services for both CHW intervention arms (high and low intensity) [96]. Wolff et al. also assessed the pre- and postintervention costs of the following services for program participants in all three intervention arms: mental and physical health, vocational and educational, residential, and supportive social [121].

Measures of effectiveness for economic analysis. Neither study created a measure of the costs per unit of program effectiveness (e.g., cost per additional day in stable housing or cost per additional day of school attendance). Instead, both studies estimated program cost savings or potential cost savings by comparing health care or social services costs in the preintervention time period with costs in the postintervention time period.

For example, the Seattle study estimated urgent care costs for the targeted children in the 2 months before the start of the intervention and compared these values without analogous costs in the 2-month period before the exit interview [96]. For this work, Krieger et al. defined urgent care costs as the costs of hospital admissions, emergency department visits, and unscheduled clinic visits [96]. Because this intervention sought to reduce use of urgent health care services among participants with asthma, a reduction in urgent care costs for participants may be viewed as cost savings attributable to the intervention.

The homelessness prevention intervention also compared preintervention and postintervention costs for participants in each of the study arms. For this work, Wolff et al. calculated costs for the following services, by study arm:

- mental health inpatient,
- mental health outpatient,
- physical health inpatient,
- physical health outpatient,
- vocational and educational,
- residential,

- cash social support, and
- in-kind social support [121].

Wolff et al. also provided a total cost amount that summed the per-patient costs for all of the above services and included the intervention cost for assertive community treatment (with or without CHWs) [121]. However, reductions in these total or specific services costs should not be viewed as cost savings attributable to the intervention because utilization and costs of some services might be expected to rise, rather than fall, as the result of a successful intervention. For example, successful assertive community treatment interventions might lead to larger pre/postintervention increases in vocational and educational service costs than a brokered case management approach.

Economic outcomes. In the Seattle program, costs for the high-intensity CHW intervention were $1,124 per child higher in 2001 dollars than costs for the low-intensity CHW intervention [96]. Estimated costs for the low-intensity asthma intervention were not provided [96].

For the homelessness prevention intervention, annual program costs were $6,200 per participant for the assertive community treatment intervention with CHWs and $6,440 per participant for assertive community treatment only [121]. These cost estimates are in 1992 dollars and are in addition to costs for brokered case management—costs that were not reported in the article. Adjusting these cost estimates to 2001 dollars using the CPI-U, we estimate the costs of assertive community treatment with CHWs to be $7,826 per patient and the costs of assertive community treatment only to be $8,129 per patient, in addition to costs for brokered case management.

For the Seattle study of children with asthma, Krieger et al. also provided estimates of pre/postintervention health care cost reductions attributable to the CHW asthma intervention [96]. Comparing urgent care costs in the 2 months before the intervention with costs in the 2 months at the end of the intervention, they estimated cost reductions of $201 to $334 per child in 2001 dollars [96]. For the low-intensity CHW group, analogous cost reductions were $185 to $315 per child. Assuming these cost reductions persist for 1 year, estimated annual cost reductions are $1,200 to $2,000 per child for the high-intensity CHW intervention in 2001 dollars. Krieger et al. also discussed the cost-effectiveness of the high-intensity intervention relative to the low-intensity approach [96]. They found savings in urgent care costs for the high intervention group relative to the low intervention group of $57 to $80 per child over a 2-month period [96]. The authors reported that if these cost reductions were to last for 3 to 4 years, the high- intensity intervention would be cost saving relative to the low-intensity intervention. Whether assuming the same level of reduced urgent care utilization and costs for several years postintervention is reasonable, however, remains unclear. The authors did find that urgent care utilization remained low in the high-intensity group for at least 6 months following the intervention [96].

For the study of homeless mentally ill participants, Wolff et al. conducted regression analyses to explore whether study arms differed in their measures of total costs over the 18-month study period [121]. They found no difference in total costs across study arms after controlling for patients' costs in the preintervention period [121]. They also compared 6-month costs in the preintervention period to 6-month costs for three separate postintervention periods (1 to 6 months, 7 to 12 months, and 13 to 18 months). At least in part because the number of participants in each intervention arm was relatively small (N = 35, 28, and 22, respectively), postintervention costs varied a great deal across time periods. The authors point out that, when comparing the preintervention period with the first 6 months' postintervention period, inpatient mental health services costs fell $1,315 for assertive community treatment with CHWs, rose almost $4,500 for assertive community treatment only, and rose more than $8,000 for brokered case management [121]. Considering the second 6-month period of the intervention, inpatient mental health services costs fell by more ($4,400 per participant) in the assertive community treatment only group than in the assertive community treatment with CHWs group ($2,651 per participant). Inpatient mental health services costs also declined in that time period for the brokered case management group ($1,252 per participant). All of these cost estimates are in 1992 dollars.

The cost estimates for health and social services that Wolff et al. [121] report are difficult to interpret using the currently recommended framework for performing and evaluating cost-effectiveness analyses [130, 131]. The recommended approach for performing cost-effectiveness analysis is to specify the perspective of the study a priori and to calculate net costs for use in cost-effectiveness evaluation as intervention costs less any costs for health care or other relevant variables (including productivity losses) averted by the intervention. The societal perspective is recommended for economic evaluation, which implies that all costs should be included, regardless of who bears them. Although the Wolff et al. [121] article implies that the intent was to estimate costs from the societal perspective, their measure of total costs excludes criminal justice and family burden costs (mentioned as a limitation), it excludes productivity costs, and it includes societal transfers (cash and in-kind support) that are not recommended for inclusion in economic analyses from the societal perspective. The presentation of costs in three different intervention time periods also makes it difficult to interpret the Wolff et al. estimates, because costs differed a great deal over time for each intervention arm [121]. Finally, the total cost measures they presented cannot readily be used in economic evaluations without some adjustments. Their total cost estimates represent the sum of intervention costs and specific health care and social services costs. These total cost estimates vary a great deal across intervention arms (including for the preintervention period) and across time within each intervention arm. In contrast, the recommended estimates for use in economic evaluations are measures of net costs that provide a single measure of costs for each intervention arm that subtract from intervention costs the health care, productivity, and other related cost reductions attributable to the intervention [131].

Economics: child health. *Study characteristics.* Two studies evaluated program costs for CHW interventions that sought to improve child health [75, 80]. One study, set in Maryland, evaluated the impact of a high-intensity CHW intervention for children with nonorganic failure to thrive in a low-income urban setting. As reported by Black et al., children diagnosed with failure to thrive were randomized to receive either the CHW intervention, which involved the delivery of clinical services plus weekly home visits from a trained CHW, or the clinical intervention only [75]. The Home Visitation 2000 RCT targeted low-income, pregnant women for a home visiting intervention that involved prenatal home visits, followed by home visits every 1 to 2 months until the target child was 2 years of age [80]. In this study, Olds et al. compared the impact of using CHWs to deliver the home visiting intervention with the impact of using nurses [80]. In addition to program costs, it evaluated several child health and developmental outcomes (e.g., mother-child interaction, quality of the home environment, child developmental outcomes).

Overview of economic analysis results. Both studies reported intervention program costs. Cost components for the failure-to-thrive trial included salaries for the CHW or nurse, materials costs, transportation costs, costs of police service, and a 10 percent overhead fee [75]. Olds et al. provided a per-family total cost of the 2.5 year Home Visitation 2000 trial [80], but they did not specify details on what was included in the cost estimate.

Measures of effectiveness for economic analysis. Because both of these studies reported only the intervention costs, they did not examine intervention costs in relationship to outcomes. Thus we had no measures of intervention effectiveness for these economic analyses.

Economic outcomes. Annual program costs for the failure-to-thrive CHW intervention were $2,828 per child in 1993 dollars [75]. Although the article did not explicitly state this, we assumed that this cost estimate reflects the additional costs of the CHW intervention relative to the clinical intervention (usual care). When adjusted to 2002 dollars using the CPI-U, the CHW intervention for these children has an estimated annual cost of $3,520 per child. For the Home Visitation 2000 and $6,162 per family for the CHW intervention arm [80]. These costs are for the full 2.5 years of the program. Dividing these estimates by 2.5, we estimate annual costs of $3,656 per family for the nurse home visitation intervention and $2,465 for the CHW home visitation intervention— both in 2002 dollars.

Table 33. Summary of economic analyses of CHW interventions

Author, Year	Intervention Description	Annual Intervention Program Costs Per Participant, Year of Dollars Specified or Assumed	Annual Intervention Program Costs, 2008 Dollars	Results of Other Economic Analyses
Stockdale et al., 2000 [22]	Mammography screening intervention	$52 (1997)	$70	$903 per additional mammography screening, 1997$ $46,308 per life-year saved for intervention plus mammogram, 1997$
Paskett et al., 2006 [17]	Mammography screening intervention	$404 (2000 assumed)	$505	$4,986 per additional mammography screening, (2000$ assumed)
Krieger et al., 2005[96]	Asthma management intervention	$1,124 (2001)	$1,366	$201-$334 reduced urgent care costs per child, high-intensity CHW intervention, 2001$
Wolff et al., 1997 [121]	Homelessness prevention intervention	$6,200 (1992) (CHW intervention)	$9,514	Reductions in inpatient mental health services costs for CHW intervention relative to usual care in all intervention time periods
Olds et al., 2002 [80]	Child health and development intervention	$2,565 (2002) (CHW intervention)	$3,070	None
Black et al., 1995 [75]	Child health intervention	$2,828 (1993)	$4,214	None

CHW, community health worker.

Economics: summary of findings. Table 33 summarizes findings from the six CHW intervention articles that provided information on program costs and other economic outcomes (presented in the order of discussion above, by clinical context). Cost estimates are shown as presented in each article, but we also report each cost estimate adjusted to 2008 dollars using the CPI-U. Although adjusting some of the cost estimates using the medical care component of the CPI might have been more appropriate, because that component accounts for faster growth in prices in the health care sector than in other parts of the US economy, we used the CPI-U because all studies relied on nonmedical labor to provide the CHW intervention.

KQ 4: Training of Community Health Workers

Characteristics of Training for Community Health Workers

Overview. *Study characteristics.* As noted in Section 2, an inclusion criterion specific to KQ 4 was that all studies reported on changes in knowledge or skills among CHWs after training. Although we identified 46 citations that were potential includes [111, 132-176], only 9 studies (10 citations) provided evidence of changes in knowledge or skills among CHWs after training [137, 141, 143, 147-150, 155, 169, 176].

All included studies were set in minority or underserved communities. Three focused on cancer prevention [137, 141, 143, 176], two on cardiovascular disease [147, 149], and one each on health promotion [169], tobacco cessation [150], salmonella prevention in the manufacture of queso fresco [155], and on health insurance enrollment, immunizations, and asthma prevention [148].

The studies included in this section spanned a variety of models of CHW interventions. Five studies relied on volunteers; [137, 141, 149, 155, 169, 176] other studies either paid CHWs or did not report on payment status. The size of the intervention effort also varied: the number of CHWs trained through these programs ranged from 4 [147] to 1,504 [148]. The educational background and prior training of the CHWs undergoing training were rarely reported: one study reported that 98 percent (of 79 CHWs) had either a college bachelor's or graduate degree [137], whereas another study reported that all trainees (4 CHWs) had 10 years of prior experience as CHWs [147]. Studies also varied in their degree of specificity in reporting eligibility criteria for CHWs. The contribution of CHWs to developing training materials varied, ranging from intensive involvement in pretesting to no involvement. Studies also varied in their reporting on training components; in the following sections, we describe reported data on components of training.

Training on cultural competence. Two studies reported training for cultural competence, but they provided no details on the content, method, and number of sessions [148, 149].

Table 34. CHW training and evaluation results

Author, Year Study Name Setting: Geography Setting: Organizational, Social, Cultural	Objective or Aim of Training	Training on Content/Health Topic	Evaluation and Testing Results of the Curriculum (Improvements in CHW Knowledge)
Balcazar et al., 2006 [149] Salud Para Su Corazon-National Council of La Raza Escondido, California; Chicago, Illinois; Ojo Caliente, New Mexico Latino communities	To promote heart-healthy behaviors among Latinos	Not described	The closed-format pre/posttest scores reported a score of 74% correct for the pretest and 100% for the posttest (n = 11). Differences in pre-post promotora knowledge score changes (N = 29) were statistically significant ($P < 0.05$) but data reported in bar graph only
Beck et al., 2007 [143] Center for Health Communities' cancer education program Milwaukee County, Wisconsin African- American churches	To train the trainer in cancer education	2 90-minute train-the-trainer workshops	Pre/post percentage correct— Ability to define cancer: General: 89/93; breast: 79/86; colon: 15/57; prostate: 80/75 Ability to identify signs and symptoms of cancer: General: NA; breast: 71/88; colon: 81/93; prostate: 40/75 Ability to identify screening recommendations: General: NA; breast 67/67; colon: NA; prostate: 80/75 Ability to identify risk factors: General: 59/85; breast: 54/92; colon: 19/89; prostate: 40/75 Ability to identify strategies to reduce cancer risk: General: 70/78; breast: 8/33; colon: 92/96; prostate: 20/75
Bell et al., 1999 [155] Abuela Project Yakima County, Washington Hispanic communities	To train Hispanic women to make queso fresco that was authentic in taste and texture but did not use raw milk in an effort to reduce the incidence of Salmonella serotype Typhimurium infections	Workshops on how to make new queso fresco recipe (i.e., without raw milk)	Pretraining/posttraining: Recognized health risks associated with eating unpasteurized milk and cheese (N): 10/14; 14/15 Make queso fresco with fresh unpasteurized milk: 6/12; 1/15.

Table 34. (Continued)

Author, Year Study Name Setting: Geography Setting: Organizational, Social, Cultural	Objective or Aim of Training	Training on Content/Health Topic	Evaluation and Testing Results of the Curriculum (Improvements in CHW Knowledge)
	resulting from eating queso fresco made from raw milk		
Kuhajda et al., 2006 [147] Pine Apple Heart Disease and Stroke Project Pine Apple, Alabama African-American women in rural southern community	To train CHWs for heart disease and stroke and in skills for counseling and assessing high-risk women in the Pine Apple clinic	Topics addressed in training included cardiovascular disease; developing action plans (heart attack, congestive heart failure, stroke); high blood pressure; tobacco control; cancer (lung, colorectal, breast, cervical)	Counseling CHWs' responses on pre/post training questionnaires showed increases in knowledge and self-reported behaviors in each of the following areas: heart disease and stroke prevention strategies, cancer prevention strategies, heart attack or stroke signs and symptoms, cancer signs and symptoms, current heart disease and stroke prevention activities, current cancer prevention activities. Data reported in bar graph only
Martinez-Bristow et al., 2006[150] Tobacco Free El Paso El Paso, Texas Neighborhood clinics	To train Spanish-speaking counselors to deliver tobacco cessation interventions	5 days of training for each level of certification for nicotine addiction	Results from pre/posttest measuring self-confidence suggest that participants understood training material; data NR Mean satisfaction scores (1 = definitely not confident to 5 = definitely confident) high for recipients of each certification: Beginner: 4.8, intermediate: 4.7, advanced: 4.6
Navarro et al., 2007 [141, 176] Por La Vida Cuidandome San Diego, California Latino communities	To train community health advisors to conduct interactive educational group sessions and train-the-trainer and their "learning partners"	Manual had sessions for understanding female body, breast cancer, Pap test, breast health, risks	Changes in knowledge and behavior, pre/post test for primary participants; and learning partners (percentage naming the following test for breast/cervical cancer early detection): BSE 58.6/74.7; 46.4/56.3 Clinical breast exam: 29.1/28.8; 28.8/20.7 Mammography: 49.8/71.2; 45.0/63.1 Pap test: 84.6/91.9; 79.3/85.1 Knows BSE: 90.5/99.3; 82.4/93.2 Knows mammography recommendations: 32.3/55.8; 27.4/38.1 Names 1 breast cancer symptom: 75.1/96.8; 70.3/94.1 Names 1 treatment for breast cancer: 40.0/65.6; 27.9/45.0 Names 1 risk factor: 8.1/16.5; 6.8/7.2 Names 1 factor for cervical cancer: 30.9/59.6; 24.3/35.1

Author, Year Study Name Setting: Geography Setting: Organizational, Social, Cultural	Objective or Aim of Training	Training on Content/Health Topic	Evaluation and Testing Results of the Curriculum (Improvements in CHW Knowledge)
			BSE in past month: 62.3/87.4; 55.9/71.5 Mammography ever: 63.3/70.0; 66.7/68.3 Pap test ever: 92.3/97.9; 88.3/92.8
Perez et al., 2006 [148] Northern Manhattan Community Voices Collaborative Northern Manhattan, New York, neighborhoods	To train community health workers, focusing on facilitating insurance enrollment, child immunization, and asthma management	Yes, but not described	Pre/post scores in competency and knowledge (gains, percentage change): Insurance enrollment: 24%/72% (gain = 48%; percentage change = 200; n tested = 61) Immunization promotion: 83%/96% (gain = 48%; percentage change = 16; n tested = 472) Asthma management: 63%/83% (gain = 20%; percentage change = 32; n tested = 499)
Williams et al., 1996 [169] No study name Atlanta and Fort Valley, Georgia Older African Americans	To raise awareness of and increase participation of older African Americans in health promotion activities	Training divided into 3 categories: G1: chronic disease education and self-care G2: lifestyle education G3: consumer education Topics for these categories developed into 12 training modules	Obtained score 80 on pre/posttest for hypertension and diabetes training sessions: Urban, low to middle income: 32%/60% Inner-city, low income: 11%/72% Rural, mixed income: 28%/93%
Yu et al., 2007 [137] No study name Southeast Michigan Chinese communities	To increase the self-efficacy of CHWs in conducting breast cancer screening promotion	Training manual had 9 sections and 5 appendices (1 was a bilingual glossary of medical terms); content includes socioedemographic characteristics and special health concerns, outreach strategies, effective communication skills for promoting screening. Also a web site, PowerPoint slides, and audio recordings available	Change in trainees' knowledge and self-efficacy Knowledge—mean number of correct answers pre (SD)/post (SD): 6 (1.4)/8 (1.1), $P < 0.001$ Self-efficacy—mean score pre (SD)/post (SD): 61.0 (11.5)/65.0 (9.2), $P = 0.016$

BSE, breast self examination; CHW, community health workers; CVD, cardiovascular disease; NA, not applicable; SD, standard deviation.

Training on recruitment and retention process skills. Two studies reported training on recruitment and retention [141, 150, 176]. One study noted that client recruitment was addressed, but the content, method, and number of sessions was not reported [150]. The other recorded five 2-hour sessions covering recruitment strategies and role-playing practice [141, 176].

Training on intake and assessment. One study reported training for intake and assessment, specifically on community mobilization, communication skills, and outreach strategies, but it provided no details on the content, method, and number of sessions [148]. A second study noted two training sessions for assessment and role-play [147].

Training on protocol delivery. Two studies reported on training on protocol delivery [147, 148]. One provided no further details [148], and the second listed health education counseling as part of the curriculum, and included role play for cancer screening counseling sessions and cardiovascular disease counseling sessions that was followed by external feedback from a clinical psychologist [147].

Training on health topic. The purpose of training CHWs on health topics was to prepare them to educate participants. Seven studies described the health content of their training in some detail; [137, 141, 143, 147, 150, 155, 169, 176] all provided evidence of change in knowledge of skills after training (Table 34). Only two reported significance tests.

Training on evaluation. A single study reported evaluation as one of the seven core modules in their curriculum but provided no further details [148].

Other training. Four studies reported training on communication skills [137, 148, 149, 176], and a single study reported on making referrals [176]. Training curricula may well have included additional elements that were not reported.

Patient Outcomes of Community Health Worker Training

We did not identify any studies that reported on patient health outcomes of CHW interventions that were linked to characteristics of training.

SECTION 4. DISCUSSION

This section discusses our findings for four key questions (KQs) relating to the interaction between community health workers (CHWs) and clients (KQ 1), outcomes of CHW interventions (KQ 2), costs of CHW interventions (KQ 3), and training of CHWs (KQ 4). As noted in earlier sections, KQs 1 and 4 are largely descriptive. KQs 2 and 3 are more analytic; they focus on health and cost-effectiveness outcomes. We specify in this discussion the strength of the evidence for the KQs related to outcomes (KQ 2) and cost-effectiveness (KQ 3); we also evaluate the applicability of studies included for outcomes (KQ 2). We refer readers to Section 2 for methods for evaluating the strength of evidence and quality of studies.

The strength of evidence for each outcome incorporates grades for risk of bias, consistency, directness, precision, and the presence of other modifying factors. Our approach is based on one developed by the Evidence-based Practice Center program for its comparative effectiveness review activities [57]. In the outcome-specific tables that follow, our overall grade of the strength of evidence appears in the far right column; grades for key domains are in the intermediate columns.

Table 35. Number of studies, by clinical focus and intensity of interventions

Primary Clinical Context	Low Intensity (percentage)	Moderate Intensity (percentage)	High Intensity (percentage)	Total Number of Studies (percentage)
Health promotion and disease prevention	2 [107, 117] (18.2)	4 [66, 69, 70, 105, 118, 119] (36.4)	5 [16, 64, 65, 67, 68, 71, 127] (45.5)	11 (100)
Injury prevention	1 [126] (33.3)	2 [101, 102] (66.7)	None	3 (100)
Maternal and child health	None	None	15 [71-87] (100)	15 (100)
Cancer screening	6 [19-22, 59, 60, 103, 104, 107, 108, 113] (40.0)	7 [15, 63, 106, 109-112, 116, 125] (46.7)	2 [17, 18, 61, 62] (13.3)	15 (100)
Chronic disease management	None	5 [23, 99, 114, 122-124] (38.5)	8 [27, 88-98, 100, 120] (61.5)	13 (100)
Total (may be less than sum of rows because of overlapping studies)	8	18	27	53

In this review, we ultimately had grades of only moderate or low. To recapitulate, moderate means that we have moderate confidence that the evidence reflects the true effect; further research may change our confidence in the estimate of effect and in fact may change the estimate. Low means that we have only low confidence that the evidence reflects the true effect; further research is likely to change the confidence in the estimate of effect and is likely to change the estimate [57].

Interactions between Community Health Workers and Clients (KQ 1)

KQ 1 asks for descriptions of the interaction between CHWs and participants; specifically, we examined place of service, type of service, type of educational materials used, duration of interaction with participants, and length of followup. We identified 53 studies with 79 citations in all, addressing KQ 1 [15-23, 27, 59-105, 107-114, 116-124, 126-128].

CHWs interacted with participants in a broad array of locations, using a spectrum of materials at varying levels of intensity. Studies usually described the place of service and type of intervention in some detail. Across the studies, one-on-one interventions generally occurred in the home, on the telephone, or in a medical setting; by contrast, group interventions tended to take place in a community setting. Studies described types of educational materials poorly or not at all. Studies inconsistently reported duration of interaction with participants and length of followup (the number and length of sessions), and they did not always clarify whether their reporting was based on protocol or on actual experience. The frequent failure to distinguish between protocol and actual experience represents a missed opportunity to explore the balance between planned and actual resource allocation and to identify strategies to translate effective CHW interventions into a variety of community settings.

Table 36. Summary of studies reporting on outcomes by primary clinical context and subtopic

Primary Clinical Context and Subdomain	Number of Studies by Outcomes					
	Knowledge	Behavior	Satisfaction	Health Outcomes	Health care utilization	Total*
Health promotion and disease prevention						
Health promotion and disease prevention: pediatric immunizations	None	None	None	3	None	3
Health promotion and disease prevention: health promotion – Latina health	None	1	None	None	1	2
Health promotion and disease prevention: disease prevention	2	5	None	1	1	6
Injury prevention						
Injury prevention: home safety	None	2	None	None	None	2
Injury prevention: workplace safety	None	1	None	None	None	1
Maternal and child health						
Maternal and child health: prenatal care and perinatal outcomes	None	None	None	5	1	6
Maternal and child health: child development	None	None	None	4	None	4
Maternal and child health: environment conducive to child well-being	None	3	None	7	None	10
Cancer screening						
Cancer screening (overall)	2	2	None	None	None	2
Cancer screening: breast self-examination	None	5	None	None	None	5
Cancer screening: Pap smears	None	None	None	None	6	6
Cancer screening: mammography	None	None	None	None	11	11

Primary Clinical Context and Subdomain	Number of Studies by Outcomes					
	Knowledge	Behavior	Satisfaction	Health Outcomes	Health care utilization	Total*
Cancer screening: clinical breast examination	None	None	None	None	4	4
Cancer screening: colorectal cancer screening	None	None	None	None	2	2
Chronic disease management						
Chronic disease management: diabetes mellitus	1	2	None	4	None	4
Chronic disease management: hypertension	None	None	None	3	1	4
Chronic disease management: infectious diseases	None	None	None	None	1	1
Chronic disease management: back pain	None	None	None	1	None	1
Chronic disease management: mental health	None	None	1	1	1	1
Chronic disease management: asthma	None	2	None	2	2	2
Total*	5	22	1	27	30	53

*Total may be less than sum of cells because of overlapping studies

We synthesized the variety of ways that CHWs can interact with participants into a single measure of intensity that serves as a proxy of resource allocation. Interactions that reported at least four of six elements suggesting a higher intensity (one-on-one, face-to-face, 1 hour per session or more, 3 or more months' duration, three or more interactions, and tailored materials) were classified as high intensity. Interventions with two or three elements were classified as moderate intensity. Interventions with only one or none of the elements of high intensity were classified as low intensity.

Of the total of 53 studies, we classified 27 as high intensity [16-18, 27, 61, 62, 64, 65, 67, 68, 71-98, 100, 120, 121, 127, 128], 18 as moderate intensity [15, 23, 63, 66, 69, 70, 99, 101, 102, 105, 106, 109-112, 114, 116, 118, 119, 122-125], and 8 as low intensity [19-22, 59, 60, 103, 104, 107, 108, 113, 117, 126].

The intensity of CHW interventions varied by clinical context (Table 35). Maternal and child health and chronic disease management interventions were all moderate or high intensity, whereas prevention and screening studies were more likely to involve low-intensity interventions.

Outcomes of Community Health Worker Interventions (KQ 2)

KQ 2 asks about the impact of CHWs on outcomes, with specific attention to the following five domains: knowledge, behavior and behavior change, satisfaction, health outcomes, and health care utilization. A key source of heterogeneity is the clinical context of the CHW intervention. The applicability of our findings is related to the clinical context of intervention. Studies targeted one or more of five primary contextual categories and a wide array of specific topic areas (number of subdomains in parentheses): health promotion and disease prevention (3), injury prevention (2), maternal and child health (3), cancer screening (6), and chronic disease management (6); collectively the focus of the studies in this review covered 20 distinct clinical or public health activities. Four studies overlapped primary clinical categories [67, 68, 71, 107].

Table 37. Effect of CHW interventions on knowledge: strength of evidence

Number of Studies; # of Subjects	Risk of Bias Design/ Quality	Consistency	Directness	Precision	Other Modifying Factors (Intensity, Confounding)	Results	Overall Strength of Evidence
Health promotion and disease prevention: disease prevention							
2; 6,841 [16, 117, 127]	Medium 1 RCT, 1 prospective cohort/fair	Consistent	Indirect	Precise	Absent	Favors CHW intervention vs. print or no intervention (for improved knowledge of label reading, knowledge of fat in diet, and knowledge of where to obtain free condoms)	Moderate
Cancer screening							
2; 1,788 [17, 18, 109]	Low 2 RCTs/1 good, 1 fair	Consistent	Indirect	Imprecise	Absent	Favors CHW vs. media or mail	Moderate
Chronic disease management: diabetes mellitus							
1; 150 [27]	Medium 1 RCT/fair	Consistency unknown (single study)	Direct	Not reported	Absent	Favors CHW intervention vs. usual care plus pamphlets (for knowledge of label reading)	Low

CHW, community health worker; RCT, randomized controlled trial.

As Table 36 demonstrates, we found numerous research gaps in the key clinical areas and domains. Satisfaction and knowledge are virtually ignored by studies in this evidence base. By contrast, health outcomes and health care utilization are better represented by studies we included; more than one-half of the studies included one or both of these outcomes.

In the section below, we discuss the strength of evidence for these five primary outcome domains and specific subdomains, reflecting the clinical context of the intervention. We follow the examination of outcomes with a summary of results for each clinical context and subdomain and then consider applicability.

We identified 53 studies comprising 79 citations addressing KQ 2. Thirty-eight were randomized controlled trials (RCTs) [16-18, 27, 61, 62, 64, 65, 67, 68, 71-98, 100, 106, 120, 121, 127, 128] and 15 were observational studies [59, 60, 71, 72, 83, 86, 87, 93-95, 102, 108, 113, 116, 117, 123, 125, 126]. Of the 53 studies, we rated 4 as good quality [17, 18, 69, 70, 96, 97, 103], 29 as fair [16, 27, 59-63, 66-68, 72, 75, 76, 79-85, 88-93, 98, 100, 101, 105, 106, 108, 109, 114, 117, 122, 124, 125, 127] , and 20 as poor [15, 19-23, 64, 65, 71, 73, 74, 77, 78, 86, 87, 94, 95, 99, 102, 104, 107, 110-113, 116, 118-121, 123, 126, 128].

Knowledge

As noted in Section 1, studies examining the effectiveness of CHW interventions are based in part on theories of individual behavior change. Studies relying on social cognitive theory as a model of individual behavior change anticipate that participants in CHW interventions will change their behavior based on knowledge they gain by observing and learning from CHWs.

Very few studies presented evidence on the effect of CHW interventions on the knowledge of participants (Table 37). The five studies reporting information on knowledge together provide (a) moderate strength of evidence that CHW interventions improve the knowledge of participants on disease prevention [16, 117, 127] and cancer screening [17, 18, 109] compared with other alternatives, (b) low strength of evidence that CHW interventions improve knowledge of label reading compared with usual care, but (c) insufficient evidence for knowledge of other issues related to the clinical or self-management of diabetes, such as dietary knowledge, appropriate diet, frequency of checking blood sugar, understanding the need for eye doctor visits, knowledge of how diabetes affects the body (eye, kidney, nerve, cardiovascular problems), or understanding insulin or other medication [27].

This literature did not compare CHWs with a comprehensive range of usual care providers. Therefore, we cannot conclude that CHWs outperform all alternatives in improving participant knowledge. Nevertheless, for the much smaller subset of comparators and outcomes included in this literature, the studies together suggest that CHW interventions can improve participant knowledge when compared with alternative approaches such as no intervention, media, mail, or usual care plus pamphlets.

We found no evidence on knowledge for all other clinical topics and subdomains, as documented above in Table 36. The absence of data on the vast majority of clinical concerns that investigators in this field sought to study (as listed in Table 36) suggests that researchers may have elected to give priority to collecting and publishing data on health outcomes and health care utilization data rather than intermediate outcomes such as knowledge.

Table 38. Effect of CHW interventions on behavior: strength of evidence

Number of Studies; # of Subjects	Risk of Bias Design/ Quality	Consistency	Directness	Precision	Other Modifying Factors (Intensity, Confounding)	Results	Overall Strength of Evidence
Health promotion and disease prevention: health promotion – Latina health							
1; 357 [64, 65]	High 1 RCT/poor	Consistency unknown (single study)	Indirect	Not reported	Present	No difference between CHW intervention and tailored or off-the-shelf interventions	Low
Health promotion and disease prevention: disease prevention							
5; 1,125 + 12 Churches [16, 67, 105, 107, 118, 119, 12]	Medium 5 RCTs/3 fair, 2 poor	Inconsistent	Indirect	Imprecise	Present	Mixed results: 3of 5 studies favor CHW intervention vs. control (no intervention, combination of interventions, media/print)	Low
Injury prevention: home safety							
2; 909 [101, 102]	Medium 2 RCTs/1 fair, 1 poor	Inconsistent	Indirect	Precise	Present	No difference between CHW and health professional or no intervention	Low
Injury prevention: workplace safety							
1;786 [126]	High 1 prospective cohort/poor	Consistency unknown (single study)	Direct	Imprecise	Present	Favors CHW over community intervention	Low
Maternal and child health: environment conducive to child well-being							
1,052 [75, 76, 78, 84, 128]	Medium 3 RCTs/2 fair, 1 poor	Inconsistent	Direct	Imprecise	Present	Mixed results: Most with no difference between CHW & control; some benefit to CHW over no intervention	Low

Number of Studies; # of Subjects	Risk of Bias Design/ Quality	Consistency	Directness	Precision	Other Modifying Factors (Intensity, Confounding)	Results	Overall Strength of Evidence
Cancer screening: planned use of screening tests							
1,612 [63, 116]	Medium 1 RCT, 1 cohort/1 fair, 1 poor	Inconsistent	Indirect	Imprecise	Present	Mixed results: 1 study shows benefit in CHW arm vs. usual, other shows no difference vs. no intervention	Low
Cancer screening: breast self-examination							
5; 3,798 [61, 62, 108, 1 10-112, 116, 125]	Medium 2 RCTs, 3 cohorts/3 fair, 2 poor	Inconsistent	Direct	Imprecise	Present	Mixed results: 2 of 5 studies show benefit of CHW vs. alternative (mail or minimal CHW), 3 of 5 show no difference vs. delayed or no intervention	Low
Chronic disease management: diabetes mellitus							
2; 213 [88-92, 124]	Medium 2 RCTs/fair	Consistent	Indirect	Precise	Absent	Favors CHW intervention vs. usual care plus newsletter	Low
Chronic disease management: asthma, use of bedding encasements							
2; 572 [96, 97, 100]	Low 2 RCTs/1 good, 1 fair	Consistent	Indirect	Precise	Absent	Favors CHW vs. less intense CHW arm or delayed CHW arm	Moderate
Chronic disease management: asthma, other behaviors (smoking cessation, removal of mold)							
2; 572 [96, 97, 100]	Low 2 RCTs/1 good, 1 fair	Inconsistent	Indirect	Imprecise	Absent	No difference between CHW vs. less intense CHW arm or delayed CHW arm	Low

CHW, community health worker; RCT, randomized controlled trial.

Behavior

Twenty-two studies reported on the effect of CHW interventions on participant behavior. The evidence for workplace safety, diabetes mellitus, and the use of bedding encasements for asthma, from five studies, suggests that CHW interventions can change participant behavior in the desired direction when compared with alternatives such as a community intervention, a lower- intensity CHW intervention, and usual care combined with a pamphlet (Table 38) [17, 18, 88-92, 96, 97, 100, 109, 124, 126]. The strength of evidence is moderate for the use of bedding encasements for asthma and low for workplace safety and diabetes mellitus.

The evidence for disease prevention, improving the environment for child well-being, planned use of cancer screening tests, and breast self-examination, from 14 studies, is mixed. Some studies demonstrate a statistically significant benefit from the CHW arm, but others show no significant differences [16, 61-63, 67, 75, 76, 78, 84, 105, 107, 108, 110-112, 116, 118, 119, 125, 127, 128]. The strength of evidence for these outcomes is low.

The evidence for health promotion among Latinas, injury prevention at home, and smoking cessation to reduce asthma, from five studies, failed to demonstrate that CHW interventions resulted in statistically significant different outcomes than alternatives; the strength of evidence for these outcomes is low [64, 65, 96, 97, 100-102]. We found no evidence to evaluate the effectiveness of CHW interventions for all other clinical concerns described in Table 36.

Together these studies suggest that CHW interventions can, in some instances, yield greater positive changes in participant behavior than a range of alternatives (including no intervention, community intervention, usual care plus a newsletter, media/print, a less intense or delayed CHW arm, or a combination of interventions). In other instances, CHWs interventions provided no statistically different benefit when compared with a range of alternatives, in the context of improvements in all arms. When the alternative requires greater resource allocation, as with the use of health professionals, the absence of a statistically significant difference may support the use of CHWs [101].

The absence of consistent evidence showing that CHW interventions provide greater benefit when compared with alternatives may be explained in part by either the inadequacy of the CHW approach in changing some behaviors or other factors such as limitations of study design and the Hawthorne effect. Regarding the effectiveness of the CHW approach, CHWs may be more effective at changing behaviors that are relatively easy to adopt (such as the use of bedding encasements provided through the intervention) and less effective in changing behaviors that may require additional support (such as smoking cessation) or more resources (such as the removal of mold or changing home environments). Study design considerations such as the choice of lower-intensity CHW interventions or the use of other fairly intensive alternatives (or both situations) may not produce statistically significant differences between the CHW arm and the alternative; the absence of differences may be further compounded by inadequate power in many of these studies. As for the Hawthorne effect, when CHWs collect or report on outcomes in all study arms (as was often the case in these studies), this lack of blinding of outcomes assessors can induce an observation-related improvement in performance.

Satisfaction

CHW interventions are often expected to prompt individual and social change and thereby reduce health disparities in either access to care or outcomes of care (or both). An indirect measure of improved access to the health care system is the participant's satisfaction with care. A single study, focusing on mental health among the homeless, found no differences between study arms in participant satisfaction; the strength of evidence for this outcome is low (Table 39).

We found no evidence to evaluate the effectiveness of CHW interventions for the other 19 other clinical concerns described in Table 36. We note that our exclusion of studies without comparison arms may have excluded program evaluations that examined participant satisfaction in greater detail.

Health Outcomes

The literature examined CHW effectiveness on a range of outcomes. Of the 53 studies, 27 reported specifically on health outcomes (Table 40).

The evidence for back pain and for improving psychosocial outcomes among caregivers of children with asthma, from three studies, provides moderate strength of evidence that CHW interventions improve health outcomes when compared with either a lower-intensity CHW intervention or a delayed-intervention control group [96, 97, 100, 114].

The evidence for seven clinical areas and subdomains—pediatric immunizations, prenatal care and perinatal outcomes, child development, environment conducive to child well-being, diabetes, mental health, and asthma symptoms—from 22 studies, is mixed. Some studies suggested that CHW interventions are more effective than alternatives (including no intervention, usual care, and nurses), but others produced no differences between CHW interventions and alternatives [27, 67-93, 96, 97, 100, 124, 128].

For disease prevention, hypertension, and mental health, the evidence from five studies suggests no difference between CHW interventions and alternative approaches, including the use of CHWs in a lesser capacity, nurses, and print materials; the strength of evidence for these outcomes is low [16, 23, 94, 95, 98, 99, 120, 121, 127]. We found no evidence to evaluate the effectiveness of CHW interventions for other clinical concerns described in Table 36.

Our overall assessment for the effect of CHWs on health outcomes is similar to our assessment of their effect on behavior change. Together these studies show that CHW interventions can have a greater effect on health outcomes than certain alternative options such as no intervention, usual care, and nurses, but these findings are not consistent across all studies; several studies find no statistically significant benefit to the CHW arm when compared with alternative approaches. The strength of evidence for the reported absence of differences is therefore low. As with our summary assessment of the effect of CHW interventions on change in participant behavior, we believe that in the context of comparable gains in study arms and the absence of statistically significant differences among study arms, the choice of CHW interventions may be reasonable when the comparator is a high-resource alternative.

Table 39. Effect of CHW interventions on participant satisfaction: strength of evidence

Number of Studies; # of Subjects	Risk of Bias Design/ Quality	Consistency	Directness	Precision	Other Modifying Factors (Intensity, Confounding)	Results	Overall Strength of Evidence
Chronic disease management: mental health							
1;165 [120, 121]	High 1 RCT/poor	Consistency unknown (single study)	Direct	Not reported	Present	No difference between CHW intervention and control	Low

CHW, community health worker; RCT, randomized controlled trial.

Table 40. Effect of CHW interventions on health outcomes: strength of evidence

Number of Studies; # of Subjects	Risk of Bias Design/ Quality	Consistency	Directness	Precision	Other Modifying Factors (Intensity, Confounding)	Results	Overall Strength of Evidence
Health promotion and disease prevention: pediatric immunizations							
3;5, 406 [68-72]	Medium 2 RCTs, 1 cohort/1 good, 1 fair, 1 poor	Inconsistent	Direct	Imprecise	Present	Mixed results: 2 of 3 studies favor CHW intervention vs. control; 1 shows no difference between CHW interventions and no intervention	Low
Health promotion and disease prevention: disease prevention							
1; 294 [16, 127]	Medium 1 RCT/fair	Consistency unknown (single study)	Direct	Not reported	Absent	No difference between CHW intervention and print intervention (for change in body mass index)	Low
Maternal and child health: prenatal care and perinatal outcomes							
5; 3,389 [71, 77, 79, 83, 86, 87]	High 2 RCTs, 3 cohorts/2 fair, 3 poor	Inconsistent	Some direct, some indirect	Imprecise	Present	Mixed results, between CHW and professionals or no intervention or usual care	Low
Maternal and child health: child development							
4;1,664 [75, 76, 78, 80-83, 128]	Medium 3 RCTs, 1 cohorts/3 fair, 1 poor	Inconsistent	Direct	Imprecise	Present	Mixed results: 2 studies show some benefit for CHW vs. no intervention or health professional, 2	Low

Table 40. (Continued)

Number of Studies; # of Subjects	Risk of Bias Design/ Quality	Consistency	Directness	Precision	Other Modifying Factors (Intensity, Confounding)	Results	Overall Strength of Evidence
						show no difference between CHW and health professional	
Maternal and child health: environment conducive to child well-being							
7; 2,299 [67, 68, 73, 74, 78, 84, 85, 128]	Medium 7 RCTs/4 fair, 3 poor	Inconsistent	Mostly indirect	Imprecise	Present	Mixed results: 5 studies show no benefit for CHW over alternatives, 2 show benefit of CHW arm vs. usual care or health professional	Low
Chronic disease management: diabetes mellitus							
4; 479 [27, 88-93, 124]	Low 4 RCTs/fair	Inconsistent	Direct	Imprecise	Absent	Mixed results: 2 of 4 studies found CHW more effective than usual care in decreasing mean HgbA1c, 2 found no difference	Low
Chronic disease management: hypertension							
3;2,823 [23, 94, 95, 9 8, 99]	Medium 2 RCTs, 1 cohort/1 fair, 2 poor	Consistent	Direct	Precise	Present	No difference between CHW intervention and CHW in a lesser capacity	Low
Chronic disease management: back pain							
1; 255 [114]	Medium 1 RCT/fair	Consistency unknown (single study)	Direct	Not reported	Absent	Favors CHW intervention vs. usual care plus a book for Roland score at 6 months and worry score at 12	Moderate

Number of Studies; # of Subjects	Risk of Bias Design/ Quality	Consistency	Directness	Precision	Other Modifying Factors (Intensity, Confounding)	Results	Overall Strength of Evidence
						months; no difference in Roland score at 12 months	
Chronic disease management: mental health							
1; 165 [120, 121]	High 1 RCT/poor	Consistency unknown (single study)	Direct	Not reported	Present	No difference between CHW intervention and usual care (health professionals)	Low
Chronic disease management: asthma symptoms							
2; 572 [96, 97, 100]	Low 2 RCTs/1 good, 1 fair	Inconsistent	Direct	Imprecise	Absent	Mixed results: 1 favors CHW vs. delayed intervention; no Difference between CHW and less intense intervention	Low
Chronic disease management: asthma, caregiver psychosocial outcomes							
2; 572 [96, 97, 100]	Low 2 RCTs/1 good, 1 fair	Consistent	Direct	Precise	Absent	Favors CHW vs. less intense CHW arm or Delayed intervention	Moderate

CHW, community health worker; RCT, randomized controlled trial.

Table 41. Effect of CHW intervention on health care utilization: strength of evidence

Number of Studies; # of Subjects	Risk of Bias Design/ Quality	Consistency	Directness	Precision	Other Modifying Factors (Intensity, Confounding)	Results	Overall Strength Of Evidence
Health promotion and disease prevention: health promotion – Latina health							
1; 103 [66]	Medium 1 RCT/fair	Consistency unknown (single study)	Direct	Imprecise	Present	No difference Between CHW and mail	Low
Health promotion and disease prevention: disease prevention							
1; 421 [105]	Medium 1 RCT/fair	Consistency unknown (single study)	Direct	Precise	Absent	Favors CHW Intervention vs. no intervention	Moderate
Maternal and child health: prenatal care and perinatal outcomes							
1; 145 [79]	Medium 1 RCT/fair	Consistency unknown (single study)	Indirect	Imprecise	Absent	Favors CHW vs. health professional	Low
Maternal and child health: Environment conducive to child well-being							
1; 730 [78, 128]	High 1 RCT/poor	Consistency unknown (single study)	Indirect	Imprecise	Present	No difference Between CHW Intervention and routine clinical care	Low
Cancer screening: Pap smears							
6; 4,366 [17, 18, 61-63, 110-112, 125]	Low 5 RCTs, 1 observational/1 good, 4 fair, 1 poor	Inconsistent	Direct	Imprecise (when reported)	Present	Mixed results: 3 of 6 studies show some difference between CHW and minimal CHW, media, direct mail, and usual care, 3 show no difference between CHW and mail or no intervention	Low

Number of Studies; # of Subjects	Risk of Bias Design/ Quality	Consistency	Directness	Precision	Other Modifying Factors (Intensity, Confounding)	Results	Overall Strength Of Evidence
Cancer screening: mammography							
11; 17,401 [15, 17-22, 59-62, 103, 104, 108, 110-113, 116, 125, 177]	Medium 6 RCTs, 5 observational studies/2 good, 4 fair, 5 poor	Consistent	Direct	Precise (when reported)	Present	8 of 11 studies favor CHW vs. no intervention, mail, print, or minimal CHW; 3 show no difference CHW and no-intervention control	Moderate
Cancer screening: clinical breast examination							
4; 3,386 [61, 62, 110-112, 116, 125]	High 2 RCTs, 2 observational/2 fair, 2 poor	Consistent	Direct	Imprecise	Present	No difference between CHW intervention and mail, CHW in lesser capacity and no intervention	Low
Cancer screening: colorectal cancer screening							
2; NR [107], 78[106]	High 2 RCT/1 fair, 1 poor	Inconsistent	Direct	NR	Present	Mixed results, 1 study favors CHW versus usual care, the other shows no difference between CHW intervention and controls (no-intervention control, tailored print and video)	Low
Chronic disease management: hypertension							
1; 722 [123]	High 1 cohort/ poor	Consistency unknown (single study)	Direct	Not reported	Present	Favors CHW intervention vs. no intervention	Low
1; 244 [122]	Medium 1 RCT/fair	Consistency unknown (single study)	Direct	Precise	Absent	Favors CHW Intervention vs. control group given	Moderate

Table 41. (Continued)

Number of Studies; # of Subjects	Risk of Bias Design/ Quality	Consistency	Directness	Precision	Other Modifying Factors (Intensity, Confounding)	Results	Overall Strength Of Evidence
Chronic disease management: infectious diseases							
						bus tokens, but monetary incentive was more effective than CHW or control given bus tokens	
Chronic disease management: mental health							
1; 165 [120, 121]	High 1 RCT/poor	Consistency unknown (single study)	Indirect	Not reported	Present	No difference Between CHW Intervention and usual care (health professionals)	Low
Chronic disease management: asthma							
2; 572 [96, 97, 100]	Low 2 RCTs/1 good, 1 fair	Consistent	Direct	Precise	Absent	Favors CHW vs. less intense CHW arm or delayed intervention	Moderate

CHW, community health worker; RCT, randomized controlled trial.

Health Care Utilization

More than half of the 53 identified studies (30 studies) reported on health care utilization (Table 41).

Fifteen studies provide moderate strength of evidence that CHW interventions increase appropriate health care utilization for disease prevention, mammography, infectious diseases, and asthma when compared with a range of alternatives such as no intervention, mail, print, or a less intense CHW arm [15, 17-22, 59-62, 96, 97, 100, 103-105, 108, 110-113, 116, 122, 177]. Two studies provide low strength of evidence that CHW interventions provide benefits in health care utilization when compared with nurses for prenatal and perinatal care and usual care for hypertension [79, 123].

For Pap smears, six studies provide mixed evidence. Some studies report statistically significant benefit for the CHW arm but others find no significant differences; the strength of evidence for this outcome is low [17, 18, 61-63, 110-112, 125]. For health promotion among Latinas, child well-being, clinical breast examination, colorectal cancer screening, and mental health, evidence from nine studies suggests that the CHW intervention and alternatives do not differ; the strength of evidence for these outcomes is low [61, 62, 66, 78, 106, 107, 110-112, 116, 120, 121, 125, 128]. We found no evidence to evaluate the effectiveness of CHW interventions for all other clinical concerns described in Table 36.

Together, these studies provide either low or moderate evidence that CHW interventions increase some appropriate health care utilization (e.g., more use of cancer screening tests, less use of emergency services) when compared with a range of alternatives for disease prevention, mammography, infectious diseases, and asthma. For other reported outcomes, however, the evidence is mixed or does not show a statistically significant benefit of the CHW arm. As with our discussion of results for participant behavior and health outcomes, we note that for some outcomes that had no statistically significant benefit of the CHW arm, the strength of evidence is low; the reasons are similar to those discussed above and include study design, choice of comparators, and the Hawthorne effect.

Applicability of Findings about Outcomes

Our analysis of applicability reviewed studies by clinical context along five dimensions: population, intensity of treatment, choice of comparator, outcomes, and timing of followup. We summarize these findings across all studies below.

Population. CHW interventions were generally conducted in underserved populations and were not overly restrictive in their inclusion criteria. We note, however, that individual studies tended to focus on a specific subset, such as low-income Latinas or inner-city African-Americans, of the larger and diverse group of the underserved. As a result, the intervention effects are likely to be applicable to the population studied, but the findings cannot be extrapolated as being relevant to all underserved populations. In particular, the applicability of these studies to low-income populations that would not qualify for Medicaid, but could not afford health insurance, is unclear.

Intensity of the treatment. As noted in earlier sections, the studies in this review were predominantly high intensity (51 percent) or moderate intensity (34 percent) rather than low intensity (15 percent). We found CHW interventions for Pap smears to be more effective than comparison efforts (such as no intervention, media, print, community interventions, and usual care) only in the relatively limited circumstances of low- and moderate-intensity interventions rather than high-intensity interventions. We found no clear evidence of variation in the effectiveness of CHW interventions by intensity of the intervention for any other outcomes. The absence of consistent evidence supporting the use of high-intensity interventions and the limited applicability of these more costly approaches to a larger population suggests that future interventions may be well served if they re-examine assumptions that high-intensity interventions work better than moderate- or low-intensity interventions.

Choice of comparator. The wide variation in the choice of comparators across all included studies reflects the immense array of options for health care in the United States. Although investigators often did justify or explain their choices of comparator, the selections often reflected a reasonable range of usual care options for the appropriate subpopulations, such as a health professional alternative for children with chronic diseases or no intervention for home safety. The diversity of these comparators does, however, limit the generalizability of our findings significantly. Our assessment of effectiveness of the CHW arm (or lack thereof) can be interpreted only in the context of the specific comparators in the literature; these findings cannot be said to be meaningful for a comprehensive range of comparators or even for usual care.

Outcomes. Forty-two percent of the 53 studies reported on behaviors, 51 percent on health outcomes, and 57 percent on health care utilization. The focus on these outcomes was appropriate and applicable to settings other than those selected for the study. The choice of outcome measures was rarely comparable across studies. The variations in outcome measures and choice of comparators precluded quantitative syntheses.

Timing of followup. Included studies by and large had an appropriate length of followup for examining the effect of the CHW intervention. Some outcomes, such as developmental outcomes for children in the relatively short term (12 months to 4 years), may not always have a high correlation with long-term health outcomes, but we regard them as appropriate for the intervention.

Summary Findings by Clinical Context

Health promotion and disease prevention. Eleven studies addressed health promotion and disease prevention, including pediatric immunizations [68-72], cardiovascular disease [105, 118, 119], diabetes prevention [16, 127]. HIV prevention [117], second-hand smoke exposure [67], colorectal cancer prevention [107], and general preventive care [64-66]. Two studies on disease prevention found that CHW interventions were more effective in changing knowledge than print or no intervention [16, 117, 127]. Results for CHW interventions on behavior outcomes were mixed, with half of the studies favoring CHW intervention versus control groups consisting of no intervention, media/print, or a combination of interventions [16, 105, 118, 119, 127]. None of the studies evaluated satisfaction outcomes. Results for CHW interventions on health outcomes, available from four studies [16, 68-72, 127], were also mixed.

The results suggest that CHW interventions can serve as an effective means of improving knowledge outcomes and possibly other outcomes related to preventing disease in underserved, minority populations.

Injury prevention. Three studies assessed injury prevention measures: two focused on home injury prevention [101, 102] and one considered workplace injury prevention [126]. The workplace study found improvements in behavior associated with CHW interventions when compared with a minimal community intervention [126] One home injury prevention study found mixed results with CHW interventions showing statistically significant benefit in some measures but controls (with no intervention) showing statistically significant benefit over CHW interventions for other measures [102]. The other home injury prevention study showed no significant difference in behavior between CHW interventions and health care professional [101]. None of the studies assessed direct health outcomes. The mixed results preclude any firm conclusions regarding the benefit of CHW interventions for injury prevention.

Maternal and child health. Fifteen studies meeting our inclusion criteria involved primarily maternal and/or child health [67, 71-87, 128]. Of these, 12 focused exclusively on potentially vulnerable populations (e.g., racial or ethnic minorities, recent immigrants, low-income families, inner-city residents) [67, 68, 71, 72, 75-77, 79-82, 84-87]. Another three targeted families identified as high risk for child maltreatment [73, 74, 78, 128] Pregnant women were part of the target population for eight studies [71, 72, 77, 79-83, 86, 87]. One study each addressed pregnant women with phenylketonuria (PKU) [83], children with failure to thrive [75, 76], and children with "chronic disease" (not otherwise characterized) [85].

Statistically significant benefit of CHWs over standard care was shown most prominently in the rapidity of metabolic control for mothers with PKU and in the mental development of infants of mothers with PKU [83]. CHW interventions were associated with a greater likelihood of initiating breastfeeding among African Americans, more frequent use of nonviolent discipline methods by parents, and higher parenting efficacy scores than either video intervention or no intervention. The study of infants with failure to thrive found a decline in cognitive and motor development among infants and an increase in depressive symptoms among mothers over time in both arms of the study; however, CHWs were significantly associated with attenuation in the decline in cognitive and motor development of infants with failure to thrive and in the increase in depressive symptoms among mothers when compared with no intervention [75, 76]. No significant advantage to CHW intervention was seen for improvements in incidence of low birth weight, presence of neonatal or infant health problems, language development, maternal stress or self- esteem, continuation of breastfeeding beyond 1 week, tobacco exposure for children of smokers, continued drug use among mothers with known prior drug use, growth of children with failure to thrive, or incidence of child maltreatment when compared with nurse interventions, multidisciplinary specialty clinical care, video or print intervention, routine health care, or no intervention.

Most studies involving CHWs for maternal and child health were concerned with high-risk populations. For maternal and child health, CHWs appear to be most beneficial when addressing existing health conditions instead of potential conditions, i.e., primary prevention. Eight of the 15 studies evaluated reported statistically significant benefit to CHWs compared with nurse interventions, multidisciplinary specialty clinical care, video or print intervention, routine health care, or no intervention. CHWs have not yet been shown to improve key health outcomes relating to maternal and child health such as prematurity, low birth weight, sustained breastfeeding, or child maltreatment relative to other alternatives such as video or print intervention, routine health care, or no intervention. The lack of such findings suggests either that further research is needed to demonstrate benefits or that the use of CHWs in this domain actually does not produce greater benefits than the use of existing approaches.

Cancer screening. Fifteen studies that examined outcomes of CHW interventions for improving breast, cervical, or colorectal cancer screening met inclusion criteria for this systematic review [15, 17-22, 59-63, 103, 104, 106-113, 116, 125]. All studies focused on minority or underserved communities. With the exception of two studies on colorectal cancer screening that included both men and women, all studies focus on increasing the rates of breast and cervical cancer screening among women.

Together, the 15 studies suggest limited evidence of improvement in knowledge in the CHW arm compared with groups receiving alternative approaches such as media or mail. Findings were conflicting about the effect of CHWs on planned or actual behavior changes, specifically breast self-examination, when compared with no intervention, delayed intervention, mail, minimal CHW, or usual care. The volume of evidence on health outcomes is limited; the quality and design of the studies limits the interpretation of available evidence.

Regarding health care utilization, our findings from limited evidence suggest that CHW interventions are not effective in comparison with other alternatives (such as no intervention, mail, tailored print and video, and minimal CHW) in raising the rates of clinical breast examination or colorectal cancer screening. More substantial evidence exists on Pap smears and mammography. It suggests that CHWs are at least as effective as alternative steps (such as mail or lower-intensity CHW interventions) in improving Pap smear rates; they are more effective than alternatives (such as no intervention, media, print, community interventions, and usual care) only in limited circumstances of low- and moderate-intensity interventions rather than high- intensity interventions. Studies demonstrated significantly greater improvements in the CHW groups than in comparison groups (no intervention, mail, print, or minimal CHW) in either the entire sample or in low-income, minority, or other underserved subsamples.

CHW interventions were more effective than alternatives (ranging from usual care to a less intense CHW arm) for increasing the appropriate use of Pap smears and mammograms, for specific subpopulations and subtypes of interventions. They were not, however, more effective than alternatives for increasing the utilization of breast self-examination, clinical breast examination, or colorectal cancer screening. CHWs can serve as a means of improving utilization of Pap smear tests and mammograms for underserved populations; the effectiveness of CHWs for other outcomes requires further research.

Chronic disease management. Thirteen studies addressed disease management for several diagnoses: diabetes mellitus [27, 88-93, 124], hypertension [23, 94, 98, 99, 123], asthma [96, 97, 100], back pain [114], mental health [120, 121], and tuberculosis [122]. Only one of these studies addressed knowledge of diabetes and found an improved score in the CHW group compared with the group receiving usual care plus educational pamphlets [27]

Two CHW interventions on diabetes [88-92, 124] and both asthma studies [96, 97, 100] addressed behavior changes; for diabetes, they favored CHW interventions over usual care and a less intense CHW arm, and for asthma, they favored CHWs with respect to improving use of bedding encasements but not smoking cessation. Only the study in mental health addressed satisfaction outcomes; it did not demonstrate a difference between the CHW and the control groups [120, 121].

Several studies investigated various health outcomes. In diabetes management, two of four studies found that a CHW intervention was more effective than usual care in decreasing HgbA1c [27, 93]. None of the four studies addressing hypertension management showed a significant difference in blood pressure control between groups [23, 94, 98, 99, 123]. Both asthma studies demonstrated that CHW interventions were effective in reducing unscheduled health care services, psychological outcomes, and behavior changes between groups [96, 97,

100]; however, symptom measures improved within the CHW and comparison groups but did not differ significantly between the groups.

In four of five studies on chronic disease management, a CHW intervention was more effective than either usual care or a less intense CHW arm in improving health care utilization for hypertension, mental health, and asthma [96, 97, 100, 122, 123]. The fifth study found that CHWs were less effective than a monetary incentive in increasing adherence to clinic appointments among tuberculosis-infected patients.

For chronic disease management, the majority of CHW interventions failed to show greater improvement in health outcomes than were observed for usual care. The exception is asthma care, for which CHWs were effective for many outcomes. Further research is necessary to determine the role of CHWs in chronic disease management.

Cost-Effectiveness of Community Health Worker Interventions (KQ 3)

Only six studies that we identified in the literature provided economic analyses of CHW interventions [17, 22, 75, 80, 96, 121]. Our analysis does not include three other studies of CHW interventions that reported information on intervention program costs but found that CHW interventions were ineffective or less effective than the baseline care approach [64, 67, 69, 70].

All six studies included for this KQ estimated intervention program costs, but not all reported the specific components of those costs or the year for which costs were estimated. Four of the studies performed economic analyses beyond program cost estimation to examine program costs in relationship to effectiveness. The two cancer screening studies both reported estimates of the cost per additional mammography screening. Although the common measures reported across these two studies suggest that comparisons might be straightforward, differences in the targeted populations nonetheless hinder comparisons of cost-effectiveness ratios across the studies. In particular, the low-intensity intervention targeted women regardless of their adherence to screening guidelines; however, the high-intensity intervention targeted only nonadherent women. The other two studies that performed additional economic analyses focused on estimating potential reductions in costs of both health care and social services attributable to the CHW intervention.

None of the CHW intervention evaluations that included an economic analysis reported a standard measure of costs per quality-adjusted life year saved as recommended in recent guides for performing economic evaluations [130, 131 2003]. One study did report on the costs per life-year saved of the CHW intervention, which is useful for comparing the intervention costs with those for other life-saving interventions, but that study provided the intervention both to women who had previously obtained mammography in line with mammogram screening guidelines and to women who had not; this approach biases the cost-effectiveness results in favor of the intervention, even when CHW time was valued using average wage rates [22]. The lack of reporting on intervention costs and cost-effectiveness according to standardized and commonly accepted measures makes it challenging to compare economic outcomes across CHW intervention studies; it also makes it even more complicated to compare cost-effectiveness between CHW interventions and non-CHW health care interventions currently being reported in the literature.

Table 42. Cost and cost-effectiveness of CHW interventions: strength of evidence

Number of Studies; # of Subjects	Risk of Bias Design/ Quality	Consistency	Directness	Precision	Other Modifying Factors (Intensity, Confounding)	Results	Overall Strength of Evidence
Health promotion and disease prevention: pediatric immunizations							
1; NA [69, 70]	---	---	---	---	---	Not evaluated because of lack of evidence of Intervention effectiveness	---
Health promotion and disease prevention: health promotion – Latina health							
1; NA [64]	---	---	---	---	---	Not evaluated because of lack of evidence of intervention effectiveness	---
Maternal and child health: child development							
2;130 [75] 630 [80]	Low 2 RCTs	Consistent	Direct	Imprecise	Absent	Cost for CHW home visitation program was lower than for nurse home visitation program; no comparison of costs to program effectiveness	Low
Maternal and child health: environment conducive to child well-being							
1; NA [67]	---	---	---	---	---	Not evaluated because of lack of evidence of intervention effectiveness	---
Cancer screening: mammography promotion							
2; 851 [17] 1,443 [22]	Moderate 2 RCTs	Consistent	Direct	Imprecise	Absent	Cost per additional mammogram is not a standardized measure that can be compared to the cost effectiveness of other interventions	Low

Number of Studies; # of Subjects	Risk of Bias Design/ Quality	Consistency	Directness	Precision	Other Modifying Factors (Intensity, Confounding)	Results	Overall Strength of Evidence
Chronic disease management: mental health							
1; 165 [121]	High 1 RCT	Consistency unknown (single study)	Direct	Imprecise	Absent	Intervention costs slightly lower for CHW arm than for traditional assertive community treatment; inconclusive results on impact of CHW on net program costs	Low
Chronic disease management: asthma							
1;170 [96]	Low 1 RCT	Consistency unknown (single study)	Direct	Imprecise	Absent	Larger urgent care cost reductions for high-intensity CHW group as compared to low-intensity CHW group.	Moderate

CHW, community health worker; RCT, randomized controlled trial.

In sum, limited evidence is currently available on the cost-effectiveness of CHW interventions for 7 of the 20 clinical contexts and subdomains we have examined in this systematic review (Table 42). For all the other clinical concerns described in Table 36, we found no evidence. Until better information is made available, assessing whether CHW interventions are a cost-effective alternative to clinical interventions to promote health and prevent disease is difficult, if not impossible.

Training of Community Health Workers (KQ 4)

We found only nine studies meeting our inclusion criteria that described the training of CHWs [137, 141, 143, 147, 150, 155, 169 148, 149, 176]. Our inclusion criterion required the evaluation of skills before and after training; all included studies reported evidence of improvement in knowledge or skills. Few studies reported on training for cultural competence, recruitment and retention process skills, intake and assessment, and protocol delivery; studies generally focused on aspects of training relevant to the health concern.

Such data are useful for future studies on the same clinical topic, but the failure to report on common elements such as cultural competence, recruitment and retention process skills, intake and assessment, and protocol delivery presents a roadblock to identifying critical elements of a standardized curriculum applicable to all CHWs. Whether studies routinely conduct such training and do not report on them is unclear from the studies that we identified.

No study reported on the effects of CHW training on health outcomes. Practitioners and policy makers seeking to institutionalize CHWs may seek to understand what measures of CHW activities best assess the effectiveness of their contributions to improved health outcomes and further, how to incorporate those elements into training curricula. As seen from the limited evidence available to answer KQ 4b, studies do not presently report sufficient information to answer this question. The question of how to tailor CHW training to improve health outcomes is a significant gap for future studies to address.

Two studies reported certification associated with their curricula. One study, focusing on tobacco cessation, offered three levels of certification: introductory ("Basic Skills to Stop Using Tobacco"), intermediate ("Treatment Specialist"), and advanced ("Leave the Addiction") [150]. A second study, on cancer education, provided a certificate of completion at the end of the training, but it gave no further details [143].

Several studies reported on the availability of their curricula for future projects. These included topics related to safe manufacture of queso fresco [155], tobacco cessation [150], breast cancer education [137], heart disease and stroke [147], and heart healthy behaviors among Latinos [149].

We note that the nine studies identified as eligible for this KQ represent a small fraction of all studies reporting on training. Other ineligible studies did not evaluate pre- and posttraining skills or knowledge: many were purely descriptive of training programs [134, 153, 154, 161, 170, 171, 175].

Among the ineligible studies that provided a critical appraisal or evaluation of the training program without pre- and posttraining results, several limited the assessment of the knowledge or skills of the CHW to the posttraining period only, without a pretest [139, 142, 145, 156, 160, 167, 173, 176]. A substantial number of other ineligible studies evaluated the training or curriculum based on feedback from designers, trainers, or other stakeholders [132,

135, 137, 138, 140, 141, 151, 152, 157-160, 162-169, 172-174, 176]. These studies could not inform our key question on training; thus, we excluded them from the systematic review proper, but we note them here to be helpful to readers who may wish to pursue these topics further.

Limitations of this Review

Limitations of the Evidence Base

Reporting. Our ability to draw conclusions on the effectiveness of CHW interventions is limited by the relative paucity of detail on specific elements of the interventions. Studies inconsistently adhered to reporting standards such as STROBE [178] and CONSORT [179], making critical appraisal of internal validity and assessment of applicability challenging. In particular, many studies did not report on the intensity of the intervention (the number and length of sessions and the time period of interaction with clients), the existence of protocols governing the intensity of intervention, or fidelity to such protocols. CHW interventions represent an opportunity to translate effective interventions into a variety of community settings; the absence of information on fidelity limits their translation. The limited available information on protocol also results in little usable data on training of CHWs.

Choice of appropriate comparators. The evidence base is marked by great heterogeneity in comparators in addition to appreciable diversity in the CHW model itself. Although appropriate comparators can and should differ by the specific outcomes being addressed, studies often did not justify the choice of comparator(s), either on its own merits or in relation to usual care. For that reason, our conclusions regarding the effectiveness of CHWs are necessarily limited. We also note that a potential Hawthorne effect may exist for studies comparing variants of CHW interventions rather than CHW interventions with usual care: the effect of the more intense arm may have been diluted by a Hawthorne effect in the less intense arm, whereby observation by CHWs could improve outcomes (at least in the short term) in the latter case.

Study design. Many studies did not report *a priori* hypotheses about their primary outcomes or give details about their power calculations (if any were done). Limited sample sizes may have resulted in studies that were not powered to find a difference between "experimental" and "control" or "comparison" groups where one may in fact exist.

A further design limitation is the frequent reliance on CHWs for data collection of outcomes in all study arms. This practice can lead to potential bias on the part of the outcome assessor; when subjects are providing responses directly to the CHWs gathering data about outcomes, their information may be colored by social desirability on their part. Moreover, a potential Hawthorne effect in this situation cannot be ruled out, as noted above.

Appropriate adjustment for confounding. The evidence base is also limited by variations in the specific confounders and effect modifiers that investigators included or controlled for in their analyses. Omitting important confounders and effect modifiers, especially co-interventions in comparison arms, limits the interpretability and utility of the evidence from such investigations. Furthermore, using the studies that did account for confounders and effect modifiers is hampered by the lack of consistent definition and inclusion of key variables.

These deficiencies together appreciably limit the consistency and validity of the evidence. As a result, we found very few outcomes for which we were able to attribute at least a moderate strength of association, despite the relatively large body of evidence that we examined.

Limitations of the Review

We limited our search to articles published in English, primarily for reasons of time and resources. We excluded studies with samples sizes less than 40. We also limited our review to the United States, so our review does not address the nature, outcomes, or cost-effectiveness of CHW interventions, or the training of CHWs, elsewhere, particularly in developing countries. However, whether CHWs in the United States have the same professional and sociodemographic characteristics as CHWs elsewhere is not well understood, so for purposes of this review, constraining the included studies to those done in the United States may not have influenced our findings much.

Our decision to include studies with comparison arms for KQs 1 and 2 likely reduced our yield of studies for knowledge, behavior, and satisfaction. We note, however, that studies reporting on knowledge, behavior, and satisfaction alone, without additional data on health outcomes, do not add to the evidence on the critical question of whether CHW interventions improve health outcomes.

For similar time and resource reasons, we did not conduct dual independent, blinded review of articles for abstraction of information into evidence tables. Instead, one reviewer performed the initial review, and a second reviewer examined that input and recommended changes or corrections when needed. These two reviewers reconciled any differences by consensus discussion. These procedures are generally in accord with the usual procedures for the RTI-UNC Evidence-based Practice Center. To enable us to address any systematic bias in our work that the above approach may have introduced, however, we did apply dual independent review for assessing the quality of individual articles and grading the strength of evidence.

The paucity of "similar" articles, for populations, patient characteristics, settings, and outcomes measured, precluded any efforts to pool findings statistically.

Future Research Directions

The evidence on CHW interventions, although extensive, could benefit from future research. We discuss methodological improvements, design considerations, and substantive gaps below.

Methodological improvements. Future studies should consistently adopt four important steps: (1) give clear conceptual models that explain the expected mechanism of change initiated by the CHW intervention, (2) justify the choices of alternative or comparison steps; (3) specify *a priori* the primary outcomes to be measured; and (4) state hypotheses that build upon the conceptual framework and the choice of comparator. In addition, studies of CHW interventions should calculate required sample size to ensure that they are adequately powered and report on those power calculations.

Studies will also benefit from external evaluation of outcomes by investigators or data collection personnel blinded to the experimental and comparison groups rather than measurement of outcomes by CHWs. Such results would be less likely to be influenced by social desirability bias or other problems of internal validity of results. These benefits must be weighed against the practical difficulties of obtaining outcome data through external observers who (unlike CHWs) may not have a relationship with the community and may be viewed with a greater degree of suspicion.

A significant gap that future studies can address is adequate reporting of design, exposures, and outcomes. Adherence to standards such as STROBE [178] and CONSORT [179] will help to improve the strength of evidence provided by this literature. More generally, studies infrequently reported the gap between planned and actual protocol delivery; reporting the changes to protocol delivery is critical to a better understanding of how to scale up effective interventions.

Design considerations. CHW interventions will also benefit from the use of practical clinical trials. CHW interventions are examples of community-based research, which is vital for successful Type 2 translation – the adaption of evidence-based interventions to real-world settings [180-182]. Representative participants, multiple and diverse settings, clinically relevant alternative interventions, and a focus on measures relevant to decision makers, which include cost, quality of life, reach, and adoption) can enhance the utility of CHW studies for translational research [183-185].

The RE-AIM framework*–reach, effectiveness, adoption, implementation, and maintenance–provides practical guidance for the development of measures of public health impact for CHW interventions [186]. Studies in our review focused on effectiveness, but they rarely provided quantitative assessments of these elements as measures of public health impact, despite their underlying reliance on models of community change in addition to individual change. Investigators may find the RE-AIM formulation helpful in providing an analytic or logic model by which to design and conduct their studies.

Substantive gaps. We identified several substantive gaps in the field that warrant further attention. They fall into several groups: (1) outcomes themselves, specifically knowledge and satisfaction; (2) clinical areas, including obesity prevention and colorectal cancer screening; (3) populations addressed, and specifically interventions for certain underserved populations; and (4) costs and cost-effectiveness analysis. We discuss these points in greater detail below.

Theoretical models underpinning CHW interventions postulate changes in knowledge as precursors to changes in behavior, health outcomes, or health care utilization. Our review uncovered surprisingly few studies that examined changes in knowledge. Although the focus on health outcomes and health care utilization is appropriate, additional evaluation of changes in knowledge would help to clarify the processes of change initiated by CHWs; such

* According to the RE-AIM framework [186] (reach is defined as the absolute number, proportion, and representativeness of individuals who are willing to participate in a given initiative, intervention, or program. Efficacy or effectiveness is the impact of an intervention on important outcomes, including potential negative effects, quality of life, and economic outcomes. Adoption is the absolute number, proportion, and representativeness of settings and intervention agents (people who deliver the program) who are willing to initiate a program. At the setting level, implementation refers to the intervention agents' fidelity to the various elements of an intervention's protocol, including consistency of delivery as intended and the time and cost of the intervention. At the individual level, implementation refers to clients' use of the intervention strategies. Maintenance is the extent to which a program or policy becomes institutionalized or part of the routine organizational practices and policies. Within the RE-AIM framework, maintenance also applies at the individual level. At the individual level, maintenance has been defined as the long- term effects of a program on outcomes after 6 or more months after the most recent intervention contact.

information would then aid investigators in refining aspects of their interventions that are not as effective as expected.

CHW interventions serve as a bridge to the health care system for the underserved and are expected to serve as a tool to reduce disparities in access to and quality of care. Improved satisfaction of participants with CHW interventions is a necessary first step to successful implementation of the intervention and eventual reduction in disparities. As with the literature on knowledge and evaluation of public health impact, single-arm studies may well report satisfaction in greater depth; more rigorous comparative studies almost uniformly do not report on satisfaction. Further investigation of satisfaction, in addition to the existing and appropriate focus on behaviors, health outcomes, and health care utilization, can help illuminate the effects of CHW interventions on health disparities.

Despite evidence of effectiveness and recommendations from a number of organizations including the US Preventive Services Task Force and the American Cancer Society, colorectal cancer screening uptake has been suboptimal. Roughly 60 percent of adults older than 50 report having been screened for colorectal cancer [187, 188]. In addition, even lower rates of screening have been reported in populations with high poverty rates [189] and in racial and ethnic minorities, including Hispanic and nonwhite populations [190]. We uncovered a single study focusing on CHW interventions for colorectal cancer; [107] future research in this area may be fruitful in identifying successful strategies for increasing screening rates for this deadly condition.

Existing CHW interventions often focus on underserved populations defined by race, ethnicity, or geographic location. Underserved groups such as low-income populations who are ineligible for Medicaid (such as low-income undocumented immigrants) and therefore at higher risk of being uninsured or the elderly may also potentially benefit from studies of CHW interventions. Important conditions for such investigators include mental health problems, dementia including Alzheimer's disease, and disabilities.

Future research on CHW interventions should focus on designing studies that prospectively collect data on program costs and effectiveness. Such work should aim to ensure that all necessary data are collected to perform and report on the cost-effectiveness or net costs of the CHW intervention as compared with baseline and alternative approaches. Program managers and local evaluators may benefit from checklists [130, 131] and step-by-step instructions for designing and performing economic evaluations of health care and community prevention interventions [191]. The first step in collecting program cost data is to list the key program activities. The next steps are to determine the perspective of the cost analysis (e.g., program, patient, or societal perspective) and to list all the resources required to support each activity (e.g., labor, contracted services, materials and supplies, building space, donated resources). The final steps are to create a system and forms for the ongoing collection of program cost data. Many resources are available to guide program managers through each step of the cost data collection process, including checklists published in Gold et al., 1996 [130] and Haddix et al., 2003 [131] and forms available online in Honeycutt et al., 2006 [191]. These lists and forms can readily be adapted to capture all of the resources used or lost in providing CHW program activities. For example, to collect and analyze the costs of multiple arms of a CHW intervention program, a list of activities and resources to support the activities should be created for each arm. Based on these lists, worksheets should be developed specific to each intervention arm for use in prospective program data collection. After all data have been collected, costs for each intervention arm should be estimated and reported alongside other study outcomes. Economic evaluations of CHW interventions should also include sensitivity analyses to examine how uncertainty or variability in assumed costs or effectiveness affects program cost-effectiveness. For example, time spent by CHWs in delivering the intervention should be given a positive value in all economic evaluations of CHW interventions, but it may also be useful to explore the extent to which valuing time at the minimum wage makes the intervention look favorable as compared with valuing time at average wage rates for paid health care workers (e.g., licensed practical nurses or medical assistants).

In summary, future economic evaluations of CHW interventions should (1) evaluate the cost- effectiveness of the interventions as compared with baseline or alternative interventions, (2) model program outcomes to estimate the program's full impact on life years or quality-adjusted life years saved to improve comparability of results, and (3) include sensitivity analyses to examine the impact of variability in economic inputs on the cost-effectiveness of CHW interventions. Using such standard approaches to evaluate CHW interventions will improve the utility and comparability of study results; thus, such approaches will also aid decision makers in determining which health promotion and disease prevention activities to support.

In the absence of consistent data on intervention costs, we created a pragmatic measure in this report to approximate the intensity of resources used for CHW interventions. Consistent data on costs in future studies will ideally provide the best information to evaluate intervention intensity. In the interim, further development and validation of pragmatic measures of resource intensity can help policy makers shape the specifics of CHW interventions to provide the most meaningful benefit for improved health outcomes.

CONCLUSION

CHW interventions have the potential to address two fundamental imperatives in improving health care in the United States: the need to address substantial and persistent health care disparities and the need to translate more research into practice. CHWs, by virtue of their role as a bridge to the health care system, can help to disseminate widely efficacious interventions to populations that rarely benefit from health care advances.

Evidence about the effectiveness of CHWs relative to other choices for providing these types of health care and public health services is at best mixed. Some studies that we assessed demonstrated statistically significant benefits of the CHW approach compared with other choices; other studies showed conflicting results or no statistically significant differences between study arms. For the latter studies, one explanation is a lack of true benefit of the CHW arm relative to other choices. In addition, the choice of controls, including health professionals and CHWs in a lesser capacity, inadequate study power, and the Hawthorne effect may explain the lack of significant differences between CHWs and alternatives.

We found limited evidence that suggests that CHW interventions can improve participant knowledge when compared with alternative approaches such as no intervention, media, mail, or usual care plus pamphlets. We found mixed evidence for CHW effectiveness on participant behavior change and health outcomes: some studies suggested that CHW interventions can result in greater improvements in participant behavior and health outcomes when compared with various alternatives, but other studies suggested that CHW interventions provide no statistically different benefits. Low or moderate strength of evidence suggests that CHWs can increase appropriate utilization for some conditions or preventive services.

The literature showed mixed results of effectiveness when analyzed by clinical context. CHW interventions had the greatest effectiveness relative to alternatives for some disease prevention, asthma management, cervical cancer screening, and mammography screening outcomes. CHW interventions were not significantly different from alternatives for clinical breast examination, self-breast examination, colorectal cancer screening, chronic disease management, or most maternal and child health interventions. We found insufficient evidence to evaluate the cost-effectiveness of CHW interventions relative to other public health interventions.

Our review suggests that CHWs may serve as a means of improving outcomes for underserved populations for some health conditions, as described above. Other health concerns require further research that addresses methodological limitations of prior studies to evaluate fully the effectiveness of CHW interventions.

REFERENCES

[1] Smith, C; Cowan, C; Sensenig, A; et al. Health spending growth slows in 2003. *Health Aff (Millwood).*, 2005 Jan-Feb, 24(1), 185-94.

[2] Moses, H; 3rd, Dorsey, ER; Matheson, DH; et al. Financial anatomy of biomedical research. *JAMA.*, 2005 Sep 21, 294(11), 1333-42.

[3] Cutler DM, Rosen AB, Vijan S. The value of medical spending in the United States, 1960-2000. N Engl J Med. 2006 Aug 31, 355(9):920-7.

[4] Arias, E. United States life tables, 2004. *National vital statistics reports.* Hyattsville, MD: National Center for Health Statistics, 2007.

[5] Agency for Healthcare Research and Quality. National Healthcare Disparities Report, 2003. Full Report. Rockville, MD: http://www.ahrq.gov/qual/nhdr03/fullreport/2003.

[6] Agency for Healthcare Research and Quality. National Healthcare Disparities Report, 2004. Full Report. Rockville, MD: http://www.ahrq.gov/qual/nhdr04/fullreport/2004.

[7] Agency for Healthcare Research and Quality. National Healthcare Disparities Report, 2005. Full Report. Rockville, MD: http://www.ahrq.gov/qual/nhdr05/fullreport/2005.

[8] Agency for Healthcare Research and Quality. National Healthcare Disparities Report, 2006. Rockville, MD: http://www.ahrq.gov/qual/nhdr06/nhdr06.htm2006.

[9] Agency for Healthcare Research and Quality. 2007 National Healthcare Disparities Report. Rockville, MD: U.S. Department of Health and Human Services, Agency for Healthcare Research and Quality; February 2008. AHRQ Pub. No. 08-0041 2008.

[10] Smedley, BD; Stith, AY; Nelson, AR. eds. Unequal treatment: confronting racial and ethnic disparities in health care. Washington (DC) Institute of Medicine: National Academies Press, 2003.

[11] Children's Defense Fund. Improving children's health: Understanding children's health disparities and promising approaches to address them. Available at <http://www.childrensdefense.org/child-research-data-publications/data/Childrens-Health-Disparities-Report-2006.pdf> 2006.

[12] Carter-Pokras, O; Bacquet, C. What is a "health disparity"? *Pub Health Rep.*, 2002, 117(5), 426-34.
[13] Health Resources and Services Administration (HRSA). Community Health Worker National Workforce Study. ftp://ftp.hrsa.gov/bhpr/workforce/chw307.pdf2007.
[14] Eng, E; Parker, E; Harlan, C. Lay health advisor intervention strategies: a continuum from natural helping to paraprofessional helping. *Health Educ Behav.*, 1997 Aug, 24(4), 413-7.
[15] Dignan, MB; Burhansstipanov, L; Hariton, J; et al. A comparison of two Native American Navigator formats: face-to-face and telephone. *Cancer Control.*, 2005 Nov, 12 Suppl 2, 28-33.
[16] Auslander, W; Haire-Joshu, D; Houston, C; et al. A controlled evaluation of staging dietary patterns to reduce the risk of diabetes in African-American women. *Diabetes Care.*, 2002 May, 25(5), 809-14.
[17] Paskett, E; Tatum, C; Rushing, J; et al. Randomized trial of an intervention to improve mammography utilization among a triracial rural population of women. *J Natl Cancer Inst.*, 2006 Sep 6, 98(17), 1226-37.
[18] Katz, ML; Tatum, CM; Degraffinreid, CR; et al. Do cervical cancer screening rates increase in association with an intervention designed to increase mammography usage? *J Womens Health (Larchmt).*, 2007 Jan-Feb, 16(1), 24-35.
[19] Derose, KP; Fox, SA; Reigadas, E; et al. Church- based telephone mammography counseling with peer counselors. *J Health Commun.*, 2000 Apr-Jun, 5(2), 175-88.
[20] Duan, N; Fox, SA; Derose, KP, et al. Maintaining mammography adherence through telephone counseling in a church-based trial. *Am J Public Health.*, 2000 Sep, 90(9), 1468-71.
[21] Derose, KP; Hawes-Dawson, J; Fox, SA; et al. Dealing with diversity: recruiting churches and women for a randomized trial of mammography promotion. *Health Educ Behav.*, 2000 Oct, 27(5), 632-48.
[22] Stockdale, SE; Keeler, E; Duan, N; et al. Costs and cost-effectiveness of a church-based intervention to promote mammography screening. *Health Serv Res.*, 2000 Dec, 35(5 Pt 1), 1037-57.
[23] Morisky, DE; Lees, NB; Sharif, BA; et al. Reducing disparities in hypertension control: a community-based hypertension control project (CHIP) for an ethnically diverse population. *Health Promotion Practice.*, 2002 04, 3(2), 264-75.
[24] Prochaska, JO; Velicer, WF. The transtheoretical model of health behavior change. *Am J Health Promot.*, 1997, 12, 38-48.
[25] Bandura, A. Social learning theory. Englewood Cliffs, NJ: Prentice Hall, 1977.
[26] Becker, MH. The health belief model and personal health behavior. *Health Educ Monog.*, 1974, 2(4).
[27] Lujan, J; Ostwald, SK; Ortiz, M. Promotora diabetes intervention for Mexican Americans. *Diabetes Educ.*, 2007 Jul-Aug, 33(4), 660-70.
[28] Perez, LM; Martinez, J. Community health workers: Social justice and policy advocates for community health and well-being. *Am J Pub Health.*, 2008, 98, 11-4.
[29] Eng, E; Parker, EA. Natural helper models to enhance a community's health and competence. In: DeCliemente R, Crosby R, Kegler M, eds. *Emerging theories and models in health promotion research and practice*. San Francisco: Jossey-Bass, 2002.

[30] Minkler, M; Wallerstein, N. Improving health through community organization and community building: a health education perspective. In: Minkler M, ed. *Community organizing and community building for health.* 2nd ed. San Francisco: Jossey-Bass 2004, 26-50.

[31] Gostin, LO; Powers, M. What does social justice require for the public's health? Public health ethics and policy imperatives. *Health Affairs.*, 2006, 25(4), 1053-60,doi:10.377/ hlthaff.25.4.

[32] Fawcett, SB; Paine-Andrews, A; Francisco, VT; et al. Using empowerment theory in collaborative partnerships for community health and development. *Am J Community Psychol.*, 1995Oct, 23(5), 677-97.

[33] Freire, P. Education for critical consciousness. *New York: Continuum International Publishing Group*, 2005.

[34] Minkler, M; Cox, K. Creating critical consciousness in health: applications of Freire's philosophy and methods to the healthcare setting. *Int J Health Serv.*, 1980, 10(2), 311-22.

[35] Kenyon, VA. Felshers and health promotion in the USSR. *Physician Assist.*, 1985, 9(7), 25-6, 9.

[36] UNICEF/WHO Management of sick children by community health workers. Accessed at<http://www.unicef.org/publications/files/Management_of_Sick_Children_by_Community_Health_Workers.pdf>on2009Feb032006.

[37] World Health Organization. World Health Statistics. Printed in France 2007.

[38] The Robert Graham Center. *Access denied: a look at America's disenfranchised.*, 2007 [cited 2-13-09], Available from: http://www.graham- center.org/online/etc/medialib/graham/documents/publications/mongraphs-books/2007/rgcmo-access-denied.Par.0001.File.tmp/rgcmo-access-denied.pdf.

[39] Wilkinson, DY. Indigenous community health workers in the 1960s and beyond. In: Braithwaite RL, Taylor SE, eds. *Health issues in the black community*. San Francisco, CA: Jossey-Bass, Inc., 1992, 255-66.

[40] Cauffman, JG; Wingert, WA; Friedman, DB; et al. Community health aides: how effective are they? *Am J Public Health Nations Health.*, 1970 Oct, 60(10), 1904-9.

[41] Kahssay, HM; Taylor, ME; Berman, PA. Community health workers: the way forward. Geneva (CH): *World Health Organization*, 1998.

[42] Minow, M. Revisiting the issues: home visiting. *The Future of Children.*, 1994, 4(2), 243-6.

[43] Boston Public Health Commission. Community Health Education Center [Internet]. Boston (MA): Boston Public Health Commission; cited 2009Feb03]. Available from <http://www.bphc.org/programs/chec/>2009.

[44] Love, MB; Legion, V; Shim, JK; et al. CHWs get credit: a10-year history of the first college-credit certificate for community health workers in the United States. *Health Promot Pract.*, 2004, 5(4), 418-28.

[45] Witmer, A; Seifer, SD; Finocchio, L; et al. Community health workers: integral members of the health care workforce. *Am J Public Health.*, 1995Aug, 85(8Pt1), 1055-8.

[46] Texas Legislative Council. House Bill 1864, enrolled version. Austin (TX): Texas Legislative Council; [last accessed February 7, 2009]. Available from: http://www.legis.state.tx.us/tlodocs/76R/billtext/h tml/HB01864F.html1864.

[47] Minnesota Session Laws 2007, Section147(HF 1078-3E). Minnesota 2007.
[48] Brownstein, JN; Bone, LR; Dennison, CR; et al. Community health workers as interventionists in the prevention and control of heart disease and stroke. *Am J Prev Med.*, 2005 Dec, 29(5Suppl1), 128-33.
[49] Norris, SL; Chowdhury, FM; Van Le, K; et al. Effectiveness of community health workers in the care of persons with diabetes. *Diabet Med.*, 2006, 23(5), 544-56.
[50] Andrews, JO; Felton, G; Wewers, ME; et al. Use of community health workers in research with ethnic minority women. *J Nurs Scholarsh.*, 2004, 36(4), 358-65.
[51] Rhodes, SD; Foley, KL; Zometa, CS; et al. Lay health advisor interventions among Hispanics/Latinos: aqualitative systematic review. *Am J Prev Med.*, 2007 Nov, 33(5), 418-27.
[52] Lewin, SA; Dick, J; Pond, P; et al. Lay health workers in primary and community health care. *Cochrane Data base Syst Rev.* 2005(1), CD004015.
[53] Gibbons, MC; Tyus, NC. Systematic review of U.S.-based randomized controlled trials using community health workers: *Johns Hopkins University Press*, 2007.
[54] Berkman, N; Viswanathan, M. Model Form for the Evaluation of Observational Studies Included in Systematic Literature Reviews. *Durham, NC: RTI International*, 2007.
[55] Deeks, JJ; Dinnes, J; D'Amico, R; et al. Evaluating non-randomised intervention studies. *Health Technol Assess.*, 2003, 7, iii-x [PMID:14499048].
[56] Downs, SH; Black, N. The feasibility of creating a check list for the assessment of the methodological quality both of randomized and non-randomised studies of health care interventions. *J Epidemiol Community Health.*, 1998, 52, 377-84.
[57] Owens, DK; Lohr, KN; Atkins, D; et al. Grading the strength of a body of evidence when comparing medical interventions: AHRQ and the Effective Health Care Program. *J Clin Epidemiol.* In press.
[58] Agency for Healthcare Research and Quality. Methods Guide for Comparative Effectiveness Reviews, Version1.0 [DraftpostedOct.2007]. Rockville, MD. Available at:http://effectivehealthcare.ahrq.gov/repFiles/2007_10DraftMethodsGuide.pdf2007.
[59] Sauaia, A; Min, SJ; Lack, D; et al. Church-based breast cancer screen in geducation: impact of two approaches on Latinas enrolled in public and private health insurance plans. *Prev Chronic Dis.*, 2007Oct, 4(4), A99.
[60] Welsh AL; Sauaia A; Jacobellis J; et al. The effect of two church-based interventions on breast cancer screening rates among Medicaid- insured Latinas. *Prev Chronic Dis.*2005 Oct, 2(4):A07.
[61] Sung, JF; Blumenthal, DS; Coates, RJ; et al. Effect of a cancer screening intervention conducted by lay health workers among inner-city women. *Am J Prev Med.*, 1997Jan-Feb, 13(1), 51-7.
[62] Sung, JF; Coates, RJ; Williams, JE; et al. Cancer screening intervention among black women in inner-city Atlanta—design of a study. *Public Health Rep.*, 1992Jul-Aug, 107(4), 381-8.
[63] Taylor, VM; Hislop, TG; Jackson, JC; et al. A randomized controlled trial of interventions to promote cervical cancer screening among Chinese women in North America. *J Natl Cancer Inst.*, 2002May1, 94(9), 670-7.
[64] Elder, JP; Ayala, GX; Campbell, NR; et al. Inter personal and print nutrition communication for a Spanish-dominant Latino population: Secretos de la Buena Vida. *Health Psychol.*, 2005 Jan, 24(1), 49-57.

[65] Elder, JP; Ayala, GX; Campbell, NR; et al. Long- term effects of a communication intervention for Spanish-dominant Latinas. *Am J Prev Med.*, 2006 Aug, 31(2), 159-66.
[66] Hunter, JB; de Zapien, JG; Papenfuss, M; et al. The impact of a promotora on increasing routine chronic disease prevention among women aged 40 and older at the U.S.-Mexico border. *Health Educ Behav.*, 2004Aug, 31(4Suppl), 18S-28S.
[67] Conway, TL; Woodruff, SI; Edwards, CC; et al. Intervention to reduce environmental tobacco smoke exposure in Latino children: null effects on hair biomarkers and parent reports. *Tob Control.*, 2004 Mar, 13(1), 90-2.
[68] Barnes, K; Friedman, SM; Brickner Namerow, P; et al. Impact of community volunteers on immunization rates of children younger than 2 years. *Arch Pediatr Adolesc Med.*, 1999 May, 153(5), 518-24.
[69] Rask, KJ; LeBaron, CW; Starnes, DM. The costs of registry-based immunization interventions. *Am J Prev Med.*, 2001 Nov, 21(4), 267-71.
[70] LeBaron, CW; Starnes, DM; Rask, KJ. The impact of reminder-recall interventions on low vaccination coverage in an inner-city population. *Arch Pediatr Adolesc Med.*, 2004 Mar, 158(3), 255-61.
[71] Barnes-Boyd, C; Norr, KF; Nacion, KW. Promoting infant health through home visiting by anurse-managed community worker team. *Public Health Nursing.*, 2001 07, 18(4), 225-35.
[72] Nacion, KW; Norr, KF; Burnett, GM; et al. Validating the safety of nurse-health advocate services. *Public Health Nurs.*, 200001, 17(1), 32-42.
[73] Barth, RP; Hacking, S; Ash JR. Preventing child abuse: an experimental evaluation of the child parent enrichment project. *J Primary Prevent.*, 1988, 8(4), 201-17.
[74] Barth, RP. An experimental evaluation of in-home child abuse prevention services. *Child Abuse Negl.*, 1991, 15(4), 363-75.
[75] Black, MM; Dubowitz, H; Hutcheson, J; et al. A randomized clinical trial of home intervention for children with failure to thrive. *Pediatrics.*, 1995 Jun, 95(6), 807-14.
[76] Hutcheson, JJ; Black, MM; Talley, M; et al. Risk status and home intervention among children with failure-to-thrive: follow-up at age 4. *J Pediatr Psychol.*, 1997 Oct, 22(5), 651-68.
[77] Caulfield, LE; Gross, SM; Bentley, ME; et al. WIC-based interventions to promote breastfeeding among African-American women in Baltimore: effects on breastfeeding initiation and continuation. *J Hum Lact.*, 1998 Mar, 14(1), 15-22.
[78] Duggan, AK; McFarlane, EC; Windham, AM; et al. Evaluation of Hawaii's Healthy Start Program. *Future Child.*, 1999 Spring-Summer, 9(1), 66-90, discussion177-8.
[79] Graham, AV; Frank, SH; Zyzanski, SJ; et al. A clinical trial to reduce the rate of low birth weight in an inner-city black population. *Fam Med.*, 1992 Aug, 24(6), 439-46.
[80] Olds, DL; Robinson, J; O'Brien, R; et al. Home visiting by paraprofessional sand by nurses: a randomized, controlled trial. *Pediatrics.*, 2002 Sep, 110(3), 486-96.
[81] Korfmacher, J; O'Brien, R; Hiatt, S; et al. Differences in program implementation between nurses and paraprofessionals providing home visits during pregnancy and infancy: a randomized trial. *Am J Public Health.*, 1999 Dec, 89(12), 1847-51.
[82] Olds, DL; Robinson, J; Pettitt, L; et al. Effects of home visits by paraprofessionals and by nurses: age 4 follow-up results of a randomized trial. *Pediatrics.*, 2004 Dec, 114(6), 1560-8.

[83] St James, PS; Shapiro, E; Waisbren, SE. The Resource Mothers Program for Maternal Phenylketonuria. *Am J Public Health.*, 1999 May, 89(5), 762-4.

[84] Schuler, ME; Nair, P; Black, MM; et al. Mother- infant interaction: effects of a home intervention and ongoing maternal druguse. *J Clin Child Psychol.*, 2000 Sep, 29(3), 424-31.

[85] Silver, EJ; Ireys, HT; Bauman, LJ; et al. Psychological outcomes of a support intervention in mothers of children with ongoing health conditions: the parent-to-parent network. *J Commun Psychol.*, 1997, 25(3), 249-64.

[86] Tessaro, I; Campbell, M; O'Meara, C; et al. State health department and university evaluation of North Carolina's Maternal Outreach Worker Program. *Am J Prev Med.*, 1997 Nov-Dec, 13(6 Suppl), 38-44.

[87] Navaie-Waliser, M; Martin, SL; Tessaro, I; et al. Social support and psychological functioning among high-risk mothers: the impact of the Baby Love Maternal Outreach Worker Program. *Public Health Nurs.*, 2000Jul-Aug, 17(4), 280-91.

[88] Batts, ML; Gary, TL; Huss, K; et al. Patient priorities and needs for diabetes care among urban African American adults. *Diabetes Educ.*, 2001May-Jun, 27(3), 405-12.

[89] Gary, TL; Bone, LR; Hill, MN; et al. Randomized controlled trial of the effects of nurse case manager and community health worker interventions on risk factors for diabetes-related complications in urban African Americans. *Prev Med.*, 2003Jul, 37(1), 23-32.

[90] Gary, TL; Hill-Briggs, F; Batts-Turner, M; et al. Translational research principles of an effectiveness trial for diabetes care in an urban African American population. *Diabetes Educator.*, 2005(6), 880-9.

[91] Gary, TL; Crum, RM; Cooper-Patrick, L; et al. Depressive symptoms and metabolic control in African-Americans with type 2 diabetes. *Diabetes Care.*, 2000Jan, 23(1), 23-9.

[92] Vetter, MJ; Bristow, L; Ahrens, J. A model for homecare clinician and home health aide collaboration: diabetes care by nurse case managers and community health workers. *Home Healthc Nurse.*, 2004Sep, 22(9), 645-8.

[93] Beckham, S; Bradley, S; Washburn, A; et al. Diabetes management: utilizing community health workers in a Hawaiian/Samoan population. *J Health Care Poor Underserved.*, 2008May, 19(2), 416-27.

[94] Frate, DA; Johnson, SA; Sharpe, TR. Solutions to the problems of chronic disease management in ruralsettings. *J Rural Health.*, 1985Jan, 1(1), 52-9.

[95] Frate, DA; Whitehead, T; Johnson, SA. Selection, training, and utilization of health counselors in the management of high blood pressure. *Urban Health.*, 1983May, 12(5), 52-4.

[96] Krieger, JW; Takaro, TK; Song, L; et al. The Seattle-King County Healthy Homes Project: a randomized, controlled trial of a community health worker intervention to decrease exposure to indoor asthma triggers. *Am J Public Health.*, 2005Apr, 95(4), 652-9.

[97] Krieger, JK; Takaro, TK; Allen, C; et al. The Seattle-King County Healthy Homes Project: implementation of a comprehensive approach to improving indoor environmental quality for low- income children with asthma. *Environ Health Perspect.*, 2002Apr, 110Suppl2, 311-22.

[98] Levine, DM; Bone, LR; Hill, MN; et al. The effectiveness of a community/academic health center partnership in decreasing the level of blood pressure in an urban African-American population. *Ethn Dis.*, 2003Summer, 13(3), 354- 61.

[99] Ward, HJ; Morisky, DE; Lees, NB; et al. A clinic and community-based approach to hypertension control for an underserved minority population: designand methods. *Am J Hypertens.*, 2000Feb, 13(2), 177-83.

[100] Parker, EA; Israel, BA; Robins, TG; et al. Evaluation of Community Action Against Asthma: a community health worker intervention to improve children's asthma-related health by reducing household environ mental triggers for asthma. *Health Educ Behav.*, 2008Jun, 35(3), 376-95.

[101] Gielen, AC; McDonald, EM; Wilson, ME; et al. Effects of improved access to safety counseling, products, and home visits on parents' safety practices: results of a randomized trial. *Arch Pediatr Adolesc Med.*, 2002Jan, 156(1), 33-40.

[102] Schwarz, DF; Grisso, JA; Miles, C; et al. Aninjury prevention program in an urban African-American community. *Am J Public Health.*, 1993May, 83(5), 675-80.

[103] Andersen, MR; Yasui, Y; Meischke, H; et al. The effectiveness of mammography promotion by volunteers in rural communities. *Am J Prev Med.*, 2000Apr, 18(3), 199-207.

[104] Fox, SA; Pitkin, K; Paul, C; et al. Breast cancer screening adherence: does church attendance matter? *Health Educ Behav.*, 1998Dec, 25(6), 742-58.

[105] Krieger, J; Collier, C; Song, L; et al. Linking community-based blood pressure measurement to clinical care: a randomized controlled trial of outreach and tracking by community health workers. *Am J Public Health.*, 1999Jun, 89(6), 856-61.

[106] Jandorf, L; Gutierrez, Y; Lopez, J; et al. Use of a patient navigator to increase colorectal cancer screening in an urban neighborhood health clinic. *J Urban Health.*, 2005Jun, 82(2), 216-24.

[107] Campbell, MK; James, A; Hudson, MA; et al. Improving multiple behaviors for colorectal cancer prevention among African American church members. *Health Psychol.*, 2004Sep, 23(5), 492-502.

[108] Erwin, DO; Spatz, TS; Stotts, RC; et al. Increasing mammography practice by African American women. *Cancer Pract.*, 1999Mar-Apr, 7(2), 78-85.

[109] Mock, J; McPhee, SJ; Nguyen, T; et al. Effective lay health worker outreach and media-based education for promoting cervical cancer screening among Vietnamese American women. *Am J Public Health.*, 2007Sep, 97(9), 1693-700.

[110] Navarro, AM; Senn, KL; Kaplan, RM; et al. Por La Vida intervention model for cancer prevention in Latinas. *J Natl Cancer Inst Monogr.*, 1995(18), 137-45.

[111] Navarro, AM; Senn, KL; McNicholas, LJ; et al. Por La Vida model intervention enhances use of cancer screening tests among Latinas. *Am J Prev Med.*, 1998Jul, 15(1), 32-41.

[112] Navarro, AM; McNicholas, LJ; Senn, KL; et al. Use of cancer screening tests among Latinas one and two years after participation in the Por La Vida Damos Cuenta program. *J Women's Cancer.*, 2000, 2(1), 23-30.

[113] Earp, JA; Eng, E; O'Malley, MS; et al. Increasing use of mammography among older, rural African American women: results from a community trial. *Am J Public Health.*, 2002Apr, 92(4), 646-54.

[114] Von Korff, M; Moore, JE; Lorig, K; et al. A randomized trial of a lay person-led self-management group intervention for back pain patients in primary care. *Spine.*, 1998Dec 1, 23(23), 2608-15.
[115] Smith, MA; Garbharran, H; Edwards, MJ; et al. Health promotion and disease prevention through sanitation education in South African Zulu and Xhosa women. *J Transcult Nurs.*, 2004Jan, 15(1), 62-8.
[116] Wilson, TE; Fraser-White, M; Feldman, J; et al. Hair salon stylists as breast cancer prevention lay health advisors for African American and Afro-Caribbean women. *J Health Care Poor Underserved*, 2008Feb, 19(1), 216-26.
[117] Wendell, DA; Cohen, DA; LeSage, D; et al. Street outreach for HIV prevention: effectiveness of a state-wide programme. *Int J STD AIDS.*, 2003May, 14(5), 334-40.
[118] Becker, DM; Yanek, LR; Johnson, WR; Jr. et al. Impact of a community-based multiple risk factor intervention on cardiovascular risk in black families with a history of premature coronary disease. *Circulation.*, 2005Mar15, 111(10), 1298-304.
[119] Cene, CW; Yanek, LR; Moy, TF; et al. Sustainability of a multiple risk factor intervention on cardiovascular disease in high- risk African American families. *Ethn Dis.*, 2008Spring, 18(2), 169-75.
[120] Morse, GA; Calsyn, RJ; Klinkenberg, WD; et al. An experimental comparison of three types of case management for homeless mentally ill persons. *Psychiatr Serv.*, 1997Apr, 48(4), 497-503.
[121] Wolff, N; Helminiak, TW; Morse, GA; et al. Cost- effectiveness evaluation of three approaches to case management for homeless mentally ill clients. *Am J Psychiatry.*, 1997Mar, 154(3), 341-8.
[122] Pilote, L; Tulsky, JP; Zolopa, AR; et al. Tuberculosis prophylaxis in the homeless. A trial to improve adherence to referral. *Arch Intern Med.*, 1996Jan22, 156(2), 161-5.
[123] Bone, LR; Mamon, J; Levine, DM; et al. Emergency department detection and follow-up of high blood pressure: use and effectiveness of community health workers. *Am J Emerg Med.*, 1989Jan, 7(1), 16-20.
[124] Corkery, E; Palmer, C; Foley, ME; et al. Effect of a bicultural community health worker on completion of diabetes education in a Hispanic population. *Diabetes Care.*, 1997Mar, 20(3), 254-7.
[125] Hiatt, RA; Pasick, RJ; Stewart, S; et al. Cancer screening for underserved women: the Breast and Cervical Cancer Intervention Study. *Cancer Epidemiol Biomarkers Prev.*, 2008Aug, 17(8), 1945-9.
[126] Forst, L; Lacey, S; Chen, HY; et al. Effectiveness of community health workers for promoting use of safety eyewear by Latino farm workers. *Am J Ind Med.*, 2004Dec, 46(6), 607-13.
[127] Williams, JH; Belle, GA; Houston, C; et al. Process evaluation methods of a peer-delivered health promotion program for African American women. *Health Promot Pract.*, 2001April1, 2001, 2(2), 135-42.
[128] Duggan, A; Windham, A; McFarlane, E; et al. Hawaii's Healthy Start Program of home visiting for at-risk families: evaluation of family identification, family engagement, and service delivery. *Pediatrics.*, 2000Jan, 105(1Pt3), 250-9.
[129] Chen, LH; Gielen, AC; McDonald, EM. Validity of self reported home safety practices. *Inj Prev.*, 2003Mar, 9(1), 73-5.

[130] Gold, MR; Siegel, JE; Russell, LB; et al., eds. Cost- effectiveness in health and medicine. *New York*: *Oxford University Press*, 1996.

[131] Haddix, A; Teutsch, SM; Corso, PS. eds. Prevention effectiveness: a guide to decision analysis and economic evaluation. *Oxford*: *Oxford University Press*, 2003.

[132] Ka'opua, LS. Training community practitioners in a research intervention: practice examples at the intersection of cancer, Western science, and native Hawaiian healing. *Cancer Control.*, 2003Sep-Oct, 10(5Suppl), 5-12.

[133] Pichert JP. Evaluating teaching skills instruction for maternal-infant health care providers. *J Nurs Staff Dev.*, 1985Fall, 1, 105-9.

[134] Robertson, EM; Franklin, AW; Flores, A; et al. African American community breast health education:a pilot project. *ABNFJ.*, 2006Jan-Feb, 17(1), 48-51.

[135] Earp, JA; Viadro, CI; Vincus, AA; et al. Lay health advisors: a strategy for getting the word out about breast cancer. *Health Educ Behav.*, 1997Aug, 24(4), 432-51.

[136] Meister, JS; Warrick, LH; de Zapien, JG; et al. Using lay health workers: case study of a community-based prenatal intervention. *J Community Health.*, 1992Feb, 17(1), 37-51.

[137] Yu, MY; Song, L; Seetoo, A; et al. Culturally competent training program: a key to training lay health advisors for promoting breast cancer screening. *Health Educ Behav.*, 2007Dec, 34(6), 928-41.

[138] LaRowe, TL; Wubben, DP; Cronin, KA; et al. Development of a culturally appropriate, home- based nutrition and physical activity curriculum for Wisconsin American Indian families. *Prev Chronic Dis.*, 2007Oct, 4(4), A109.

[139] Reinschmidt, KM; Chong, J. SONRISA: a curriculum toolbox for promotores to address mental health and diabetes. *Prev Chronic Dis.*, 2007Oct, 4(4), A101.

[140] Dick, RW; Manson, SM; Hansen, AL; et al. The Native Tele health Outreach and Technical Assistance Program: a community-based approach to the development of multimedia- focused health care information. *Am Indian Alsk Native Ment Health Res.*, 2007, 14(2), 49-66.

[141] Navarro, AM; Raman, R; McNicholas, LJ; et al. Diffusion of cancere ducation in formation through a Latino community health advisor program. *Prev Med.*, 2007Aug-Sep, 45(2-3), 135-8.

[142] Kelly, PJ; Lesser, J; Peralez-Dieckmann, E; et al. Community-based violence awareness. *Issues Ment Health Nurs.*, 2007Mar, 28(3), 241-53.

[143] Beck, B; Young, S; Ahmed, S; et al. Development of a church-based cancer education curriculum using CBPR. *J Health Care Poor Underserved.*, 2007 Feb, 18(1), 28-34.

[144] Olney, CA; Warner, DG; Reyna, G; et al. Medline Plus and the challenge of low health literacy: findings from the Colonias project. *J Med Libr Assoc.*, 2007Jan, 95(1), 31-9.

[145] Han, HR; Kim, KB; Kim, MT. Evaluation of the training of Korean community health workers for chronic disease management. *Health Educ Res.*, 2007Aug, 22(4), 513-21.

[146] Bergland, JE; Heuer, L; Lausch, C. Diabetes lay educator case study: one woman's experience working with the Hispanic migrant and seasonal farm workers. *J Cult Divers.*, 2006Fall, 13(3), 152- 7.

[147] Kuhajda, MC; Cornell, CE; Brownstein, JN; et al. Training community health workers to reduce health disparities in Alabama's Black Belt: the Pine Apple Heart Disease and Stroke Project. *Fam Community Health.*, 2006Apr-Jun, 29(2), 89-102.

[148] Perez, M; Findley, SE; Mejia, M; et al. The impact of community health worker training and programs in NYC. *J Health Care Poor Underserved.*, 2006Feb, 17(1Suppl), 26-43.

[149] Balcazar, H; Alvarado, M; Hollen, ML; et al. Salud Para Su Corazon-NCLR: a comprehensive promotora outreach program to promote heart- healthy behaviors among Hispanics. *Health Promot Pract.*, 2006Jan, 7(1), 68-77.

[150] Martinez-Bristow, Z; Sias, JJ; Urquidi, UJ; et al. Tobacco cessation services through community health workers for Spanish-speaking populations. *Am J Public Health.*, 2006Feb, 96(2), 211-3.

[151] Kim, S; Flaskerud, JH; Koniak-Griffin, D; et al. Using community-partnered participatory research to address health disparities in a Latino community. *J Prof Nurs.*, 2005 Jul- Aug, 21(4), 199-209.

[152] Smith, A; Christopher, S; McCormick, AK. Development and implementation of a culturally sensitive cervical health survey: a community-based participatory approach. *Women Health.*, 2004, 40(2), 67-86.

[153] Hansen, LK; Feigl, P; Modiano, MR; et al. An educational program to increase cervical and breast cancer screening in Hispanic women: a South west Oncology Group study. *Cance rNurs.*, 2005Jan-Feb, 28(1), 47-53.

[154] Morris, LA; Ulmer, C; Chimnani, J. A role for Community Health Corps members in youth HIV/AIDS prevention education. *J Sch Health.*, 2003Apr, 73(4), 138-42.

[155] Bell, RA; Hillers, VN; Thomas, TA. The Abuela Project: safe cheese workshops to reduce the incidence of Salmonella typhimurium from consumption of raw-milk fresh cheese. *Am J Public Health.*, 1999Sep, 89(9), 1421-4.

[156] Meyers, AR; Lett, S; Grigg-Saito, D; et al. Health care in the United States: a course for refugee health workers. *Am J Public Health.*, 1989Aug, 79(8), 1051-2.

[157] Hatch, JW. Outreachin Chatham County. *NC Med J.*, 1987Dec, 48(12), 633-5.

[158] McElmurry, BJ; Swider, SM; Grimes, MJ; et al. Health advocacy for young, low-income, inner- city women. *Adv Nurs Sci.*, 1987Jul, 9(4), 62-75.

[159] Salber, EJ. Where does primary care begin? The health facilitator as a central figure in primary care. *Isr J Med Sci.*, 1981Feb-Mar, 17(2-3), 100-11.

[160] Bullock, K; McGraw, SA. A community capacity- enhancement approach to breast and cervical cancer screening among older women of color. *Health Soc Work.*, 2006Feb, 31(1), 16-25.

[161] Teufel-Shone, NI; Drummond, R; Rawiel, U. Developing and adapting a family-based diabetes program at the U.S.-Mexico border. *Prev Chronic Dis.*, 2005Jan, 2(1), A20.

[162] Littleton, MA; Cornell, CE; Dignan, M; et al. Lessons learned from the Union town Community Health Project. *Am J Health Behav.*, 2002Jan- Feb, 26(1), 34-42.

[163] Edgren, KK; Parker, EA; Israel, BA; et al. Community involvement in the conduct of a health education intervention and research project: community action against asthma. *Health Promot Pract.*, 200507, 6(3), 263-9.

[164] Duthie, P; Philippi, E; Schultz, J. Collaboration for training: a partnership to improve quality, consistency and cost-effectiveness of essential training for community health workers. *Am J Health Educ.*, 200503, 36(2), 113-6.

[165] Castaneda, X; Clayson, ZC; Rundall, T; et al. Promising outreach practices: enrolling low- income children in health insurance programs in California. *Health Promot Pract.*, 200310, 4(4), 430-8.

[166] Ramos, IN; May, M; Ramos, KS. Fieldaction report. Environmental health training of promotoras in colonias along the Texas-Mexico border. *Am J Public Health.*, 200104, 91(4), 568-70.

[167] Maurana, CA; Rodney, MM. Strategies for developing a successful community health advocate program. *Family Community Health.*, 200004, 23(1), 40-9.

[168] Kash, BA; May, ML; Tai-Seale, M. Community health worker training and certification programs in the United States: findings from a national survey. *Health Policy.* 2007, 80(1), 32-42.

[169] Williams, MP. Increasing participation in health promotion among older African-Americans. *Am J Health Behav.*, 199611, 20(6), 389.

[170] Valverde, M; Felderman-Taylor, J. HIV/AIDS outreach in southern New Mexico: from design to implementation. *JHIV/AIDS Social Services.* 200607, 5(2), 55-71.

[171] White, JA; Drechsel, J; Johnson, J. Faithfully fit forever: a holistic exercise and wellness program for faith communities. *J Holist Nurs.*, 200606, 24(2), 127-31.

[172] Hardy, CM; Wynn, TA; Huckaby, F; et al. African American community health advisors trained as research partners: recruitment and training. *Fam Comm Health.*, 200501, 28(1), 28-40.

[173] Johnson, RE; Green, BL; Anderson-Lewis, C; et al. Community health advisors as research partners: an evaluation of the training and activities. *Fam Community Health.*, 200501, 28(1), 41-50.

[174] Zuniga, L; Ramos, G; Williams, DM. Promotora training as a preparation for entry into the work force. *Tex J Rural Health.*, 2000, 18(1), 30-4.

[175] Madigan, ME, Smith-Wheelock, L; Krein, SL. Healthy hair starts with a healthy body: hair stylists as lay health advisors to prevent chronic kidney disease. *Prev Chronic Dis.*, 2007Jul, 4(3), A64.

[176] Navarro, AM; McNicholas, LJ; Cruz, M; et al. Development and implementation of a curriculum on cancer screening for small groups of Latino women. *J Cancer Educat.*, 2007, 22(3), 186-90.

[177] Rauscher, GH; Earp, JA; O'Malley, M. Relation between intervention exposures, changes in attitudes, and mammography use in the North Carolina Breast Cancer Screening Program. *Cancer Epidemiol Biomarkers Prev.*, 2004May, 13(5), 741-7.

[178] von Elm, E; Altman, DG; Egger, M; et al. The Strengthening the Reporting of Observational Studies in Epidemiology (STROBE) statement: guidelines for reporting observational studies. *J Clin Epidemiol.*, 2008Apr, 61(4), 344-9.

[179] Altman, DG; Schulz, KF; Moher, D; et al. The revised CONSORT statement for reporting randomized trials: explanation and elaboration. *Ann Intern Med.*, 2001Apr17, 134(8), 663-94.

[180] Glasgow, RE. Translating research to practice: lessons learned, areas for improvement, and future directions. *Diabetes Care.*, 2003, 26, 2451-6.

[181] Woolf, SH. The meaning of translational research and why it matters. *JAMA.*, 2008Jan 9, 299(2), 211-3.

[182] Sung, NS; Crowley, WF; Jr. Genel, M; et al. Central challenges facing the national clinical research enterprise. *JAMA.*, 2003 Mar12, 289(10), 1278-87.

[183] Glasgow, RE; Emmons, KM. How can we increase translation of research in to practice? Types of evidence needed. *Annu Rev Public Health.*, 2007, 28, 413-33.

[184] Glasgow, RE; Klesges, LM; Dzewaltowski, DA; et al. The future of health behavior change research: what is needed to improve translation of research in to health promotion practice? *Ann Behav Med.*, 2004Feb, 27(1), 3-12.

[185] Tunis, SR; Stryer, DB; Clancy, CM. Practical clinical trials: increasing the value of clinical research for decision making in clinical and health policy. *JAMA*., 2003Sep24, 290(12), 1624-32.

[186] Glasgow, RE; Vogt, TM; Boles, SM. Evaluating the public health impact of health promotion interventions: the RE-AIM frame work. *Am J Public Health*., 1999Sep, 89(9), 1322-7.

[187] Whitlock, EP; Lin, JS; Liles, E; et al. Screening for colorectal cancer: a targeted, updated systematic review for the U.S. Preventive Services Task Force. *Ann Intern Med*., 2008Nov4, 149(9), 638-58.

[188] Centers for Disease Control and Prevention (CDC). Use of colorectal cancer tests—United States, 2002, 2004, 2006. *MMWR*., 2008, 57, 253-8.

[189] Schootman, M; Jeffe, DB; Baker, EA; et al. Effect of area poverty rate on cancer screening across US communities. *J Epidemiol Community Health*., 2006 Mar, 60(3), 202-7.

[190] Meissner, HI; Breen, N; Klabunde, CN; et al. Patterns of colorectal cancer screening uptake among men and women in the United States. *Cancer Epidemiol Biomarkers Prev*., 2006Feb, 15(2), 389-94.

[191] Honeycutt, AA; Clayton, L; Khavjou, O; et al. Guide to analyzing the cost-effectiveness of community public health prevention approaches. Prepared for the Assistant Secretary for Planning and Evaluation (ASPE)http:// aspe.hhs.gov/ health/reports/ 06/ cphp a/report.pdf) 2006March.

In: Community Health Workers
Editor: Cecilia Hodges

ISBN: 978-1-63485-060-5

Accompanying CD-ROM Table of Contents

Index

D

E

F

G

H

I

K

L

M

N

O

P

Q

R

S

Y

Z